BIODYNAMICS OF OSTEOPATHY

Phase Two

Second Edition

James Jealous D.O.

For more information about Dr. Jealous please visit:
https://BiodynamicsOfOsteopathy.com

BIODYNAMICS OF OSTEOPATHY Phase Two

Hardback ISBN: 979-8-2955-3899-5

Second Edition 2025

James Jealous D.O. (1943–2021) practiced as an osteopathic physician, teacher and writer for many years. His life's work was to found and develop the specific methodology of Biodynamics of Osteopathy, following the lineage of Dr. A.T. Still and Dr. W.G. Sutherland.

This is one of a series of Biodynamics of Osteopathy books. They grew organically from sets of handouts written by Dr. Jealous and given to students during courses taught by him and his teachers. After many years he collected the handouts together and created individual course manuals, which he added to and rewrote many times. After several more years they evolved further into books.

TABLE OF CONTENTS

OSTEOPATHY IS SERVICE

We use our hands ...

To treat the Whole patient

To listen to the indwelling movements of Life

To treat all levels of illness

To assist in building the patient's functional reserve

To support homeostasis and trophicity by balancing the activity of the autonomic nervous system

To explore "laws not framed by human hands" (Dr. Still and Dr. Sutherland)

To cooperate and communicate with the Laws of Nature (Dr. Wales)

"To find the Health" (Dr. Still)

To get to the treatment plan

To get to the diagnosis

To help establish a point of Rest or Neutral around which the Whole can come to balance

To find Cause

We believe ...

We have an innate capacity to heal

The patient functions as a whole

The autonomic nervous system plays a major role in disease and healing

Structure and function are one form of activity

The Divine is indwelling

Life moves beyond death

There is a Constant Movement toward Normal

We are here to Serve Humanity

Normal is ...

"A sense of peace and harmony" (Dr. Sutherland)

Ease of motion, without tension

A capacity for Neutral

A sense of Wholeness to Life

The capacity for adaptation, change without compensation.

"Skill is proportionate to one's understanding of normal" (Dr. Still)

BIODYNAMICS OF OSTEOPATHY, PHASE TWO

1. What defines a lesion?
2. Name two methods of creating balanced membranous tension.
3. Describe two events that usually change while waiting for a patient's neutral.
4. Describe the normal "tone" of the cerebellum.
5. Describe the activity on the transverse axis of the cerebellum during inhalation.
6. Discuss the location of the cerebellum at birth in relation to the occiput lobes and what changes you expect over the next twenty years.
7. What forces must one appreciate in order to successfully "control" a CV4?
8. Can you sense ventricular motion consistently? Describe any difficulties.
9. If you have felt a seizure threshold, describe the "feel" of it.
10. Where is the fulcrum for the involuntary motion of the sciatic nerve?
11. What is the real or theoretical relationship between central nervous system motion and neurotrophic function?
12. Specifically describe augmentation within primary respiration.
13. Can you sense "sutural disengagement" before the bones move?
14. Have you read "The Tour of the Minnow"?
15. Discuss the observer from your experience.
16. Are you consciously evaluating synchronization? Example, please.
17. What information is most useful in assessing the treatment of intraosseous lesions in children?

PRESTO!

All of my mentors who were with Dr. Sutherland from 1935 to 1954 loved to recall Will's story about the balance scale.

Dr. Sutherland was visiting with some of his friends on Cape Cod, near where Anne Wales lived. They went into a country store. Hanging from the ceiling was a replica of an old balance scale used for weighing dry goods. Will spotted it. He began a lesson right there.

He pointed out the point of suspension for the function, the fulcrum around which it came to rest, the point where the power of the function is located. Power is the capacity for rest.

As he said, "Think how little touch it takes to shift the balance scale," a wind came through the open doorway. The scales fluttered and became still again. He was delighted!

This is a story of many doorways to understanding the skills used to communicate with Primary Respiration. This is Balanced Fluid Tension. This is what it feels like when fluid is neutral and it shifts to a new point of balance. It is a suspended automatically shifting fulcrum that allows the lesion to return to Balance. When it does shift, it comes to a stillpoint of rest and reserve.

Try to imagine this story and see how many principles of treatment are between the lines.

How long does the shift take? ... Presto! And then a return of the function to balance, which takes longer.

The Balance Point is established during the Embryonic Period of your life.

I have had both eyes open all the time

To find a defect in nature's work,

Its plan, its object, its specifications,

Its building, and its engineering;

So far I have failed to find

A variation from perfection.

A. T. Still

PHASE ONE REVIEW

Phase One was a transition into Biodynamic principles.

We studied:

The thread of the Health in the lesion field

The Tissue Motion Present in the lesion with which one can omit the process of Motion Testing

The Direction of Ease

Neutral as a Prerequisite to Treatment

Neutral as an indwelling point of Rest—that is the entry point of the therapeutic forces into a lesion field

The incredible knowledge that WGS demonstrated when he noted that the lamina terminalis is the fulcrum of central nervous system motion

The evaluation of the CNS motions

The sutures as doorways that open and let the bones breathe (transmute) into the space that is created for them by the opening

The wholeness of motion ... from the center to the periphery and from the periphery to the periphery at the same time

The lesion field and motion present in the fluid, synchronizing with the inhalation pattern of Motion Present in the Fluid; we called this Balanced Fluid Tension, or BFT

Zone A, Zone B, and Zone C

PHASE TWO OVERVIEW

Phase Two is about the Fluid Body's behavior at 2–3 cpm.

Other rates and dynamics exist. We will study these activities during other Phases.

The fluid is not fluid like water; it is protoplasmic.

Protoplasm can be seen as the first moldable substance that can hold an image. Protoplasm is a magical substance, as it can become any form or function.

The Fluid Body, or Zone B, is our name for the Wholeness of the fluid functions.

The Fluid Body functions as a single drop ... (WGS).

The Fluid Body expresses growth, development, regeneration, and healing from the Potency or Power of the Tide. It is present in us throughout life.

The bodily fluids are pieces of the whole protoplasmic Fluid Body.

The Intelligence guiding the Fluid Body is not the central nervous system. This Intelligence creates the central nervous system. The Fluid Body can lesion. Becoming "locked up," it loses its capacity for Neutral and self-correction.

When it locks up, it feels like tissue or bone.

Sutherland found methods of correcting dysfunctions of the Fluid Body by restoration of its capacity for Neutral. He called the first one CV4. The method is called resuscitation.

There are pauses, Stillpoints, and Neutrals in the activity of the Fluid Body.

Once Neutral is reestablished, the Fluid Body will self- correct; this is called Automatic Shifting.

MEDITATION

Meditation Is Practicing Truth

The word "soma" is very old. It comes from Sanskrit. In my understanding it means the perfect form. Zone A is not the Soma. Zone A is the unresolved, that which cannot come into "Neutral within the Whole."

Soma is the Health. It is said that its roots are in the River of Life.

We can practice sensing the Health in ourselves by dividing our attention.

***

Anytime you wish to sense the perfect form of the Health, it's good to bear in mind that it is not as concrete as you see in anatomy books. It is much more fluent and transparent. Let it demonstrate its truth to you rather than imagining "something."

As you sense the Health, do not change your posture. Just be ordinary and sense the perfect form. Divide your concentration between Zone A and the Health.

The Health will not be on the same midline as your Zone A; it may appear to be displaced. It is not displaced; Zone A is.

***

One minute is a long time if the concentration is poised.

Spend time with the Health and your sense of the density in Zone A will change. You will be surprised how much changes with so little effort.

***

The Health has a heart. A higher Mind is indwelling there. We are not an empty house, and we do not own the property. We are a guest that is received with joy.

Protoplasm:

The First Moldable Substance That Can Hold an Image

THE FLUID BODY

The Fluid Body is Zone B. It is separate from the Health because when the whole patient lesioned, Zones A and B were formed as compensation.

The Fluid Body is not water, it is protoplasm. As you study protoplasm you will be awed by its Intelligence and how little we know about it.

There is a very interesting video available on YouTube called *Seifriz on Protoplasm – Full Film*. It was made in 1954 by William Seifriz, professor of botany at the University of Pennsylvania.

Dr. Sutherland is credited with discovery of the Fluid Body, although he never used the term himself. He said, "The fluids can lesion." This sentence changed the history of how we think about treatment and diagnosis.

We will begin our studies with sensing the Fluid Body at work. This will help us to cooperate and communicate with it. The central nervous system does not control it. The Fluid Body creates the central nervous system.

This fact makes us realize that the Fluid Body has a higher Intelligence than that of the brain. This is a hard reality in today's world, as the brain has come to be regarded as God. I assure you it is not.

Embryology has validated much of what Drs. Still and Sutherland observed and interfaced with during treatment. I believe it is best to move into the actual interface with the Fluid Body in practical sessions, and discuss theory as we mature in our skills.

***

Below are some references from authorities that need slow and concentrated digestion.

Dr. Sutherland made hundreds of comments about fluid. A review of all his writings is a big task, but it will serve you well. He had an amazingly inquiring mind. One quote that will be helpful in Phase Two is "At the balance point of the fluids you have an unerring potency." There are three elements to explore here.

1. The balancc point in the fluid. This is like the balance point of tissue, only more fluent.
2. Unerring.
3. Potency. Potency in our work refers to the power to transmute the unresolved lesions in the patient. This power replaces the clinician's own force and willpower during treatment.

Dr. Wales wrote about management of the fluids in the 1953 *OCA Journal.* She states: "Synchronize with the motion of the fluids or you will disturb them." This is vital. Synchronization as applied here means to sense, to listen to the motion of the breathing of the fluids. Within this afferent event, fluids are free to work and demonstrate their truth. If one just grabs the head and does not listen, the fluids become disturbed and the rate of the breathing increases. The fluids then cannot be seen clearly because of the turbulence. How we listen is the key. Being afferent and not efferent with our proprioception is a big lesson in life, as well as the conditioner of clinical outcomes. We must study how our own mind works to see what her teaching implies.

Dr. Magoun, in his second edition of *Osteopathy in the Cranial Field,* mentions that "the fluids have self-preservation forces." This is much the same as what Dr. Wales was pointing toward. The Fluid Body is watching our relationship with it, but the observer is not in the central nervous system. This raises some questions about the Intelligence of the Fluid Body and its cause.

Dr. Blechschmidt, the noted embryologist, in his book *Biokinetics and Biodynamics of Human Differentiation,* says the fluid fields are decisive, biokinetic (Sutherland called this Automatic Shifting), biodynamic (a mysterious outside cause not framed by genetics), and unerring in its perfect timing and formations. His descriptions fit with Sutherland's commentaries.

Dr. DeHaan, another noted embryologist, describes fluid fields as having "unerring power."

Dr. Becker describes the fluids as having "dynamic beauty." I believe his language elevates the character of the Fluid Body to a higher level than central nervous system function, as a vehicle for healing.

Dr. Schooley, in his article on fulcrums published in the 1953 *OCA Journal,* said of the fluid that it "enters the space of the fluid world with a respect for its Supreme Intelligence."

None of these men were promoting anything but were merely reflecting on what their science unveiled ... The similarities are inviting us to explore, as we will in Phase Two.

OBSERVATION OF SELF-CORRECTING FLUID FORCES

Practical

Hold your wrist in full flexion; take it to a barrier that is painful.

This strains the tissues and the Fluid Body.

Wait.

Release the wrist and let it rest in a Neutral position.

Have a partner hold the wrist and listen to what is transpiring.

What forces are working to correct the strain?

Rebalance the patient.

REBALANCING

Practical

Gently let the cranial bowl sit in your hands. Be afferent and listen. The cranial bowl sits in your hands, the hands are listening, the attention is passive: not looking into the patient, but receiving proprioception ... then images form in your mind.

Now notice Zone A and Zone B, by dividing your attention evenly between them.

Is Zone A inside Zone B, or is Zone B inside of Zone A?

Sense Zone B without any sense of Zone A ... one drop of fluid.

The bowl is transparent to the Tide. Can you see something passing through the bowl and out? Is the bowl of water breathing smoothly with one motion, or is it disturbed? If you feel that the fluid could be more at ease, then go to the Stillness in the fluid and wait. Balance is a point where the fluids breathe around a single fulcrum as one drop.

Balance should reconvene quite easily. In some cases, rebalancing is a complete treatment, especially in children.

THE SACRAL WATERBEDS

The language here is not poetic. The sacrum is suspended in two rivers of life that suffuse it: Thoracic and Primary Respiration.

We rarely see this, for two reasons. It takes a really healthy system to express it, and we do not have a vivid enough picture of normal. We project structure onto function.

The sacrum comes from fluid (protoplasm and mesenchyme) and does not begin to have bony cells for a year after birth. It is a sea of fluid that has beautiful tidal motions from both Thoracic and Primary Respiration. When it lesions, the fluid locks up and a Zone A forms. This makes the sacrum feel hard and immobile.

Today, we are training our minds to see fluid dynamics and to treat lesions without engaging tissue ease or barrier, only the fluid fields. This will hopefully demonstrate the healing power of the Fluid Body and help us see that structure alone does not exist in the body.

First let's look at the Fluid Fields that we can easily observe.

FLUID

Imagine fluid in the following spaces:

The sacral Zone B . . . where it begins, and from where it heals
The sacral and coccygeal segments
The midline of function for the sacrum
The "fluid" L5/S1 disc space
The synovial fluid-filled facets, L5/S1
The sacroiliac joints
The sacrococcygeal joint

EVALUATION AND TREATMENT OF SACRAL FLUID DYNAMICS

The normal sacrum has two basic kinds of involuntary motion: the action expressing Thoracic Respiration and the action expressing Primary Respiration. First we will evaluate for these involuntary motions, as well as the structural pattern.

Evaluation:

Biomechanical ... Structural alignment. Active palpation.

Functional ... Involuntary motion in response to Thoracic Respiration. Passive listening.

Biodynamic ... Involuntary motion in response to Primary Respiration. Afferent listening.

Any involuntary motion present is called Motion Present (see Phase One).

You should now have three pictures of sacral dynamics. Remember them, as they are important for follow-up.

THE TREATMENT OF SACRAL FUNCTION USING THE FLUIDS

After your evaluation, begin treatment as follows:

Synchronize with the breathing of Primary Respiration.

When your mind is settled, notice the points of the sacral waterbeds as described. Is any of the fluid, in any of the compartments, open and moving?

Find the space that is most "open." Go into that space and find the Motion Present in the fluid and synchronize with its inhalation activity.

Once you begin treatment, watch all the pockets of fluid ... They will all respond to what you are doing. One of the other pockets will open, so you will move with the change to the new area ... This will repeat itself until the whole fluid field reorganizes.

The fluid pockets merge as the anatomical boundaries fall away, until one fluid field remains. It feels like a pool of water. The pool becomes greater than the space of the sacral anatomy. This pool is a local Zone B that has become Neutral.

Now, wait.

A therapeutic force will enter the Neutral pool of the local fluid, and the whole of the Zone B in the whole patient will enter the treatment and go still.

Now, motion returns to the lesion field ... Reevaluate.

Rebalance if necessary.

All the pockets are really one Fluid Body working to correct itself... this will become clearer as your perception rebuilds itself.

FALSE FULCRUMS

This commentary is about the principles of sensing fulcrums within the fluid. As we know, the cerebrospinal fluid has many characteristics, including a fluctuation response along a long axis, a fluctuation response along a transverse axis, multiple spiraling movements, and a "fluid drive" that appears during the therapeutic process. We can also follow the pattern of "health" within the fluid in order to help us locate a neutral synchronistic with the Tide itself. Most of these concepts are familiar and I have only one comment to make at this moment.

It is not uncommon for practitioners to slightly compress the fluid without being aware that they are. By doing so, one can mistakenly follow the fulcrum of the reaction of the fluid to the compression. This detour can take a great length of time, be unproductive, and go "flat" at the end point, leaving the observer unclear about exactly what is happening within the mechanism. What happens in these circumstances is that one is tracking bile's own forces within the fluid, the forces that were unwittingly introduced into the fluid by the practitioner. These misinterpretations occur because one is creating a dynamic within the fluid rather than following the healing process at work.

A simple principle of treatment may "cure" this tendency, which all of us have at one time or another experienced. The method that I have found successful is for the observer to place the hands on the body and simply allow the Tide to pass through the hands, allowing the hands to act as a permeable membrane. One is in contact with the fluid, and there is an awareness of the tidal forces moving through the fluid and through the hands. Not down the hands, not into the hands, but actually passing through the hands like X-rays. One perceives the Tide and the fluid simultaneously. By dividing the attention between the Tide and the fluid, one can clearly perceive any force introduced into the fluid. This, of course, avoids creating the false fulcrums, which we could easily follow into what appears to be a therapeutic process, the end result of which is not a therapeutic process but bewilderment. Distinguishing these processes can lead one's perception to other events as well.

IATROGENIC INFLUENCES ON THE HEALING OF THE PATIENT

First, one must say that we are all human and that the perfect treatment is an ideal that may never be actualized. One hopes and behaves as if there will be a miracle "just around every turn of the Tide," and there is.

Self-ridicule is destructive and a function of the ego, disguised as humility, which in itself is neutral and not self-degrading. We are all beginners ... believe me. This discussion is to help us observe our own influence on the natural and Divine expressions of Life.

When Anne Wales was over one hundred and still treating ... she always rebalanced the patient because, as she said, "One cannot give the perfect treatment." Rebalancing, as you know, is an act of making sure one's footprints are not left on the inner landscape of the living organism.

We are learning to cooperate with the indwelling therapeutic forces that are millions of years old and organized by a Supreme Intelligence that will adjust our perception to what we can understand in the moment. The Tide gives us the perception to engage in the physician/patient interface.

It is reckless to forget this and add force or intention from one's own motive.

During any time with the patient, and especially during "hands-on," one is well advised to do the following:

1. Watch the whole patient and not just the part highlighted in one's awareness.
2. Watch the autonomic nervous system for disturbance.

3. Listen to your conscience, which is an indwelling awareness, intrinsic to the movement of the River of Life and the present moment.

There is a wonderful story in *Winnie the Pooh* in which Pooh and Piglet go hunting and nearly catch a Woozle ... After a snowy night, Piglet steps outside his Beech Tree residence to find Pooh Bear walking in circles around the tree. Piglet is curious and asks Pooh what he is doing ... Pooh says he is tracking something that he cannot see but he wants to catch up with whatever is making the tracks ... Pooh shows Piglet the tracks. Piglet thinks it must be a Woozle that Pooh is tracking. Piglet joins Pooh, and after they circle the tree, Pooh says, "Now there are two of them ... whatever it is we are tracking has been joined by another." The story continues until there are twelve sets of tracks. Christopher Robin comes and Pooh sees what he has been doing ... tracking his own footprints.

It is very possible to track our own footprints and believe we are watching a treatment.

For example:

If one is efferent and palpating the tissues without appreciating the physiology directly, then this orientation makes the fluid fluctuate in an attempt to reduce the compression. The operator thinks the fluid waves are a treatment and follows them, causing augmentation, and then it really looks like a treatment when in fact it is a footprint caused by the operator ... the sympathetic nervous energy crescendos and either goes unnoticed or is assumed to be from the patient's own anxiety. This can easily be proven.

To prevent such mishaps, we teach perceptual studies and rate relativity during the courses. The institution of afferent "listening with the hands" is essential. Later one becomes a neutral observer, allowing the Tide more "room" to be creative. Eventually, the attention is an effect of the Tide, and the treatment is generally quite short as the asynchrony is minimized. One always checks to see if rebalancing is appropriate. We can insult the soma or the fluid or the "fluid in the fluid" ... the latter two are not something we often think about very deeply because we think they are unconscious biological fields. They are not.

They are watching the immediate environment.

Sutherland demonstrated that the fluid could lesion and lock down the soma (bones). Without nerve endings, how do the "fluids" perceive us? What kind of a brain does it have? Is the fluid more intelligent than the brain? Let's think about what kind of observer the fluid is, that it precognitively senses our mental activity and tries to protect the organism from our unconscious invasive actions.

WHAT MANNER OF LESION ACTIVITY DO WE NOTICE AT DIFFERENT TIMES IN THE FLUID?

1. Static ... the fluid locks down and will not breathe, fluctuate, or transmute.
2. Aberrant fluctuations ... the fluid breaks away from the influence of the midline and demonstrates rapid lateral fluctuations that are not relating to the midline. This is a kind of bracing to prevent "fluid collapse" and flaccidity.
3. Rate shifts ... the rate of Primary Respiration shifts with the stress placed upon it. Remember that Magoun's model promoted a rate of 8–14 cycles per minute, which we now believe to be an effect of direct action palpation, that challenges the Fluid Body's health.
4. Hypersensitivity ... some patients are sensitive to palpation that is efferent, which causes the fluid to break down into pieces and also causes autonomic distress. It is our job, not the patient's, to be able to avoid this aggravation.
5. Decoys ... the psychological attention of the patient can intentionally create direction in the fluids that the operator can misinterpret as a therapeutic wave. This form of cleverness is a neurosis that needs to be understood and not challenged. In treatment, one goes around or under this pattern. Unwinding in the soma is a form of this disturbance that has been promoted by some schools. My opinion is that the unwinding reinforces the neurosis at a deeper level, while giving the patient a sense of "doing."
6. Autonomic storms ... there are many causes of autonomic overload, from post-traumatic stress to side effects from pharmaceuticals ... one must feel the high-frequency vibration and search for the cause.

7. Physical trauma ... being tossed about by an accident creates false midlines, and the Fluid Body shifts to a new axis and malfunctions.
8. Chemical toxicity/stasis ... All drugs are potentially toxic. That is why side effects are part of the physiological action of drugs. Individual responses vary, and the Fluid Body can help the physician decide what the drug is doing to the overall physiology of the patient. Any remedy can lock up the fluid, including natural or homeopathic preparations. Radiation is another source of injury that needs to be addressed.
9. Disease ... most diseases affect the Fluid Body. Diabetes, for example, causes sluggishness in the fluid due to high osmolarity. Eventually, if you keep good notes, you will find that the Fluid Body can be approached as part of the diagnostic landscape in the patient, with considerable accuracy.
10. Iatrogenic ... clinicians are mostly unaware of transmitting negative input to the patient, and yet it is rare that it does not happen. The tempo of the Tide is the only pure reference point for our actions. This truth is gracious and merciful, so one should not fear one's humanity but rather attempt neutrality to one's limits, and the pauses will smooth out the rest. Iatrogenic lesions commonly arise from the following:
    a. Conceptual brevity ... coming too quickly to a conclusion or action.
    b. Going deep ... one can miss the interface of the Tide with the patient. We like to go deep, as we think erroneously that the treatment will be more complete and whole. This use of personal preference will ultimately be at the expense of completeness and wholeness. One must be aware of one's preferences and be neutral to one's desire for familiar territory.
    c. Transparency of the hands to the motion of the Tide.
    d. Leaving the ground.

e. Not releasing the attention when the therapeutic force retires.
f. Not allowing the background to move into the foreground, by clinging to motion in the foreground.
g. Talking about the psyche when the fluid is still.

The above information is from personal notes and 45 years of research based upon exploration of Osteopathic teachings, from our tradition and the physiological principles of embryology.

"Skill is proportionate to one's understanding of Normal."

A. T. Still

NORMAL

When we are in the present moment, we are in eternity. –C. S. Lewis

Enter the fluids through the Stillness, or you will disturb them. –A. Wales

There are self-preservation forces in the fluids. –H. Magoun Sr.

The metabolic fields are decisive, intelligent, and have perfect geometry. –E. Blechschmidt

The fluids have an extra-genetic, biodynamic influence that expresses development. –E. Blechschmidt

The fluids never miss the perfect geometric intersect. –R. DeHaan, embryologist

The fluids express dynamic beauty. –R. Becker

The fluids are a continuum ... with the "Supreme Intelligence." –T. Schooley

It takes thirty-six and one-half hours for a lesion to set up a pattern after the shock and seventy- two hours for it to resolve after successful treatment. –A. Becker

Get the fluids going first, then address the soma if necessary. –R. Day

WILLIAM G. SUTHERLAND

Our tradition is vitalized by individuals who gave up knowledge for a relationship with Life. The perceptual journey into a landscape of laws not framed or conceived by human reason requires one to see with a fresh freedom. Freedom comes from finding something to relate to, out of love and adoration. Still and Sutherland both found principles and laws that were not about controlling a treatment or one's own being, but about serving a higher wisdom as it flowed into creation. As a result, much of what our teachers report seems backwards from a more Newtonian or even Quantum perspective.

The fluids can lock up; they can lesion, and when they do, the soma becomes rigid. These words seem backwards in many ways … is it not the tissues that lesion and impede the flow of the fluids? Are cranial lesions not boney somatic dysfunctions, thus mechanically impeding physiology? …

Sutherland draws us away from this thinking and presents a unique insight.

After much travail, Sutherland describes the phenomena of normal Fluid Body dynamics: he finally describes exactly the same processes as Blechschmidt did. Briefly stated, the fluid fields are metabolic continuums that are biodynamic, i.e., integrated and designed by extra-genetic environmental influences (the Tide). These metabolic actions are geometrically patterned and aligned by these same tidal forces, and are capable of biokinetic activity (Automatic Shifting) and realignment.

The position of any part is a function of the movement of the whole and is mediated by the metabolic fields, which carry the form into an integrated functional syncytium. Sutherland called this observable process "transmutation," a word that defies rational analysis. Interestingly, Carl Jung used the same words when describing the functions of the human psyche and healing.

"Unerring potency" are words Sutherland and his students used with a sense of reverence when speaking about the self-correcting forces visible to the trained eye in therapeutic events, seen when Neutral was present or established in the patient. Unerring means having perfect performance ...

Sutherland, Blechschmidt, and many others have described these perfect forces as generative or formative in nature ... The great British Osteopath Littlejohn refers to formative forces in some of his writing. Clearly one is called to explore these forces and evaluate their role in practice ... not theoretically but in relationship to the Osteopath and the patient, in the present moment, as healing is being used to engage the indwelling therapeutic forces that Still founded the profession upon.

Sutherland discovered axial fluctuations that organize the metabolic fields and the Fluid Body. He discovered a means of communication that allowed fluctuations to normalize the function of the fluid fields and allow the interchange of all the bodily fluid in a return to the continuum of wholeness.

Our task is to try to understand the principles expressed by our teachers who have worked in this manner. We must build our own relationship with life and humbly apply the principles to discover personally if they can be effective in a family practice setting.

Volumes could be written on this subject, but they would only distract us from meeting the principles directly and becoming real students of the Master Mechanic of Life.

SELF PRESERVATION FORCES

Practical

This practical exploration begins with an appreciation of the self-preservation forces present in each of us and how to listen to their guidance during treatment.

1. Four to five persons per table: one clinician, one patient, two or three observers.
2. The patient participates.
3. Synchronize with the "Breathing of Primary Respiration."
4. Adjust all voltages in all the hands to match.
5. Note the emergence of Neutral (everyone).
6. The clinician attempts to be so subtle that it cannot be detected by others.
7. Discussion.
8. Rebalancing by the clinician, as others note the point when it is done.
9. New clinician and patient.

DYNAMIC NEUTRAL

Growth, Healing, and Evolution Occur Through a Dynamic Neutral

***

Communication inside the fluid body is less than 1 mm Hg of pressure…

maybe less than zero.

Our task is to find this communication with our hands.

***

Look at the interior surface of a cranial bone. There are grooves. How do they form?

***

Space Opens and Function Moves In.

MEDITATION: FINDING ONE'S NEUTRAL

(2–3 Cycles per Minute)

We have lost our understanding of Neutral and its essential place in our lives ... a place of rest and refreshment.

Neutral is necessary for Mother Nature to keep us in balance as a growing organism. If we do not rest, we will falter ... we will become bored, anxious, stubborn, lonely, and fatigued ... even ill.

How many illnesses can be resolved by expressing one's Neutral, which allows resynchronization with the Health and healing?

Phase Two is about the activity of the Fluid Body at 2–3 cpm. A healthy Fluid Body at 2–3 cpm can express Neutral and self-correct most dysfunctions as they occur.

It's like gardening ... you aerate the earth, irrigate with plenty of water, shelter it from extremes, and feed it ... A healthy garden makes its own remedies from the soil. Good soil is self-renewing (i.e., self-composting) ... but the soil must rest, go fallow, then it can resume activity and productivity. When fallow (neutral), wholeness is restored.

Neutral reclaims Wholeness.
Thoracic Respiration can be a doorway to Neutral.
We will be observing the breathing of Thoracic Respiration.

Sit or lie in a position of ease.

Sense the whole of Zone B ... that is, the Fluid Body from below your feet to above your head ... a zone with little tension. This feels more like space than tissue.

Settle into the sensation of quiet fluid.

Divide your attention quietly to "see" your breathing and Zone B... what area in your body moves first in the function of breathing?

As the air comes up into the nose, there is a sensation that travels to the lamina terminalis ... watch the Whole and this first step of breathing...

What moves next?... The pyramidalis muscle, just above the pubes ... Then? ...

The pelvic floor releases and the pelvic bowl opens.

This creates space for the diaphragm to move downward with ease.

Just watch the cycles of your breathing.

Let your system respond as it wishes.

Do not make an effort to relax; it will happen naturally.

The autonomic nervous system will quiet.

Breathing will come to a balance point, then Neutral.

Your body (Zone A) will change density.

Thoracic and Primary Respiration will move close to one another.

Space opens and function moves in.

FLUID FLUCTUATIONS

Dr. Sutherland's perception became a vehicle for discovery. Ruby often spoke, as did Rollin, about Will's patience. He would sit and watch the "Mechanism" for long periods of time without activity. We need to be able to just watch with a neutral mind. Out of his love and discipline came a flood of observations about the nature of the fluids. He made major discoveries, the content of which require reading again and again. He spoke about fluctuations of the cerebrospinal fluid and of the Whole Fluid Body (my words).

He described a Longitudinal Fluctuation, a Lateral Fluctuation(s), and a fluctuant movement in the Whole. We will begin with the Longitudinal Fluctuation. It is not the Long-Tide.

The Longitudinal Fluctuation only occurs at 2–3 cpm. I have not been able to appreciate it at slower rates.

Dr. Sutherland recognized certain natural laws at work in the fluids that became dependable as diagnostic landmarks and therapeutic doorways to rebuilding function when the Fluid Body is lesioned. The Longitudinal Fluctuation is altered when the Fluid Body lesions. Restoration occurs when the Fluid Body goes to Neutral and then reorganizes itself and expresses a normal Longitudinal Fluctuation.

The normal pattern of the Longitudinal Fluctuation is synchronized with the inhalation and exhalation of Primary Respiration at two to three cycles per minute. The inhalation pattern is inside the patient and the exhalation movement is outside in Zone B.

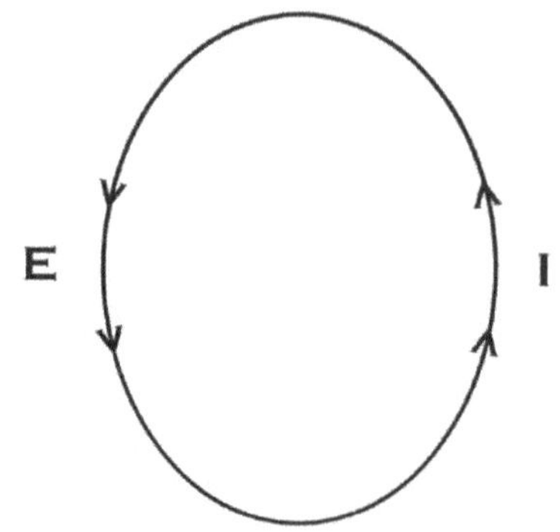

The Inhalation Pattern

At the beginning of the inhalation phase, the Longitudinal Fluctuation begins at the coccyx and slowly, over 12 seconds, raises upward in a space the diameter of a quarter. After a while it arrives at the foramen magnum. When it enters the cranium, it changes shape and cascades upward from the posterior to the middle to the anterior cranial fossa. It seems to end at the lamina terminalis.

The pattern follows the shape of the central nervous system from the tip of the coccyx to the lamina terminalis. This suggests that it may carry the original image of the CNS and that one of its functions is repatterning of the CNS. This may be why Sutherland thought it was a fluctuation in the cerebrospinal fluid, which we now see differently.

The Exhalation Pattern

After the disappearance of the inhalation movement at the lamina terminalis, the movement continues along the floor of the anterior cranial fossa and exits the soma into Zone B. If Zone B is damaged, there will be no exhalation movement of the Longitudinal

Fluctuation. If Zone B is normal (which is rare), the flow will leave the cranium near the glabella and flow in an arc along Zone B's surface and enter the midline of the notochord at the coccyx, at the end of the exhalation period.

This completes the spherical course ... It ends where it begins.

It is rare to see a normal, because the patient would have to have soul/spirit/body unification nearing wholeness at this level. Most people express only a small exhalation pattern that dies just after leaving the head.

Comments

The inhalation pattern follows the notochord. This suggests an orientation to the notochordal midline in some fashion.

The fluid fluctuations are not fluids. They are electromagnetic fields in the fluid. Sutherland called this "energy" a "fluid in the fluid" because it moved through the fluid without resistance by the fluid itself.

When one "directs the Tide," one is engaging this fluid in the fluid. This is also called the potency. Notice it is spelled with a small *p*, which distinguishes it from the Potency referring to Omnipotence and the Supreme Intelligence of the Tide.

Notice: There is potency and a Potency, a tide and a Tide, in the language we use.

Sutherland's language is confusing, but as he discovered more, he had to clarify a great deal. He had to reuse some language that he had used on smaller events to describe larger events that he discovered later. Magoun did not help to make this clear.

DIAGNOSTICS CONCERNING THE LONGITUDINAL FLUCTUATION

Alterations in the Longitudinal Fluctuation of the Fluid Body 2–3 cycles per minute

Fluctuation Is Absent ... Potency Is Held in the Coccyx:

- Sexual abuse
- Forced confinement
- Severe emotional abuse
- Mental dissociation ... "spaced-out persona"

Absent Fluctuation with No Potency in the Coccyx ... Burned-Out Ignition:

- Cocaine use, even infrequently
- Denied chemical abuse, even smoking
- Chemotherapy
- Radiation therapy
- Steroid use, more than three weeks

Fluctuation Partially Ascends and Stops:

- Self-indulgence, willfulness
- Rigid psychological boundaries
- Chronic illness
- Grief

Decreased Amplitude:

- Fatigue ... lack of rest!

Acute illness

Medications

Alcohol

Long axis compression

HIGH-AMPLITUDE LATERAL FLUCTUATION IN THE HEAD

This kind of head feels "great" ... all kinds of power, but if you look carefully, there is no longitudinal fluctuation. When a system decompensates, the longitudinal becomes weak. If the insult continues, the longitudinal shuts down and the lateral fluctuation begins to try to hold the Fluid Body together ... But the lateral fluctuation is only in the head, nowhere else. This is not a healthy situation.

The above comments are about situations I observed repeatedly in certain kinds of cases. There was a diagnostic parallel between the state of the longitudinal fluctuation and the history of the case—even though the chief complaint was not any of the things listed above.

There were many other lesion types of the Longitudinal Fluctuation; for example, paradoxical motion. In paradoxical motion, the fluctuation is inverted, going downward ... I could not assign any specific diagnostics to this kind of pattern except perhaps chronic melancholy. Once I got an email about a Longitudinal Fluctuation that was "backwards" or paradoxical.

The treatment is simple. Synchronize with the pattern of the motion of the fluctuation during inhalation, even if it is strange. The system will self-correct unless the cause is still operating.

CENTRAL STILLNESS

The skill of rebalancing becomes more refined as we see the Wholeness of the Fluid Body.

The Fluid Body is not water ... It is, as I have said many times, protoplasm. It reacts quite differently than water.

It is "one drop" ... with no anatomy.

It does not perceive distance within itself.

It grows as a singularity and heals as one unsegmented function.

Rebalancing can be done from the feet ... Throughout Phase Two we will rebalance from the feet.

Practical

Hold the feet or any part of the leg.

Sense the Fluid Body as a Whole.

Is it breathing as a Whole or are there irregularities? If so, rebalance by ...

Going to the Central Stillness ... and waiting, without distraction, in the Stillness.

Central Stillness is not at geometric center ... It is the stillness that suffuses the whole Fluid Body and is central to its existence.

FLUID BODY LESIONS

1. Dr. Sutherland was very clear in his observations of the Fluid Body and made the profound discovery that the Fluid Body could lesion and could be reoriented and revitalized through being taken to Neutral.
2. A normal Fluid Body fills Zone A and Zone B. This creates a sense of shelter for the organism. Any form of stress causes a reaction in the Fluid Body, i.e., it lesions. It can lesion in the following patterns:
    a. It can lock up as a whole (shrink).
    b. It can lose its longitudinal fluctuation and its fluid drive. It's important to remember that the longitudinal fluctuation and the fluid drive are necessary for the self-correcting process to occur.
    c. It can change its rate.
    d. It can become stiff or floppy.
    e. It can create compensatory fluid waves that can be mistaken for Automatic Shifting, which is very misleading to the observer.
3. Getting the Fluid Body to Neutral unlocks its potential power so that it can self-regulate, i.e., automatically shift.

THE FLUID CAN LESION

The history of the discovery of the Fluid Body is revealing.

I believe that reading the complete works of Dr. Sutherland is essential. There are many oversimplifications about fluid dynamics. Reading Sutherland's words is an ongoing call to a deeper understanding of the relationship of Primary Respiration to growth, development, and healing. The time allotted here, in these courses, is not designed to give you a foundation, but to build upon knowledge of his work.

"The fluids can lesion" (WGS).

This sentence changed the history of Osteopathy. What does this mean? What are the consequences of this in clinical practice? What does this sentence do to the words *anatomy, structure, junction, form,* and *lesion*? What does it mean with regard to correction of postural lesions? To our understanding of tissue restrictions? ... The Osteopathic lesion itself, does it change our understanding of its organizational forces? How does this relate to the growth and treatment of children? What skills are needed to relate to the Fluid Body?

What is its material content? How does it relate to the neuroendocrine immune system?

What integrates it? When does it appear and disappear from life processes? ... Can one sense this in oneself? ... How is it related to the body, soul, spirit?

As we pass through the Phases and do our private study, these and many other questions will appear, and you will begin to formulate an understanding. It is not an easy journey because our consciousness and language must shift if we are to see the clinical results Sutherland proposed.

THE AVAILABLE MOTION PRESENT IN THE LESION.

Synchronize with the breathing of the Fluid Body.

Find the Direction of Ease of the Reciprocal Tension Potency.

Make a decision in favor of a CV4 or EV4.

Follow the RTP in the Direction of Ease.

It will pour itself into the ocean of the Dynamic Stillness, either at the center or the periphery.

Once it has a therapeutic direction, release your attention.

The therapeutic direction may shift.

Release your attention!

Eventually the RTP returns to its birthplace (the Ocean).

As it returns, there is a Stillness that begins to maturate through and around the patient.

This may last for some time ...

Wait.

Longitudinal Fluctuation returns slowly.

Wait.

When the fluctuation is stable, with the same amplitude for three cycles, remove your hands during the inhalation phase.

Reflect on any changes within the fluid in the fluid and the Fluid Body as a result of the treatment.

Let the patient rest as long as necessary.

Rebalance the whole.

OPERATOR-INDUCED LESIONS

Zone B is larger than Zone A. Looking inside the skin for the Fluid Body compresses the outer boundary of Zone B. This will cause fluctuations that could be mistaken for therapeutic activity. Following these fluctuations is following one's own footprints. One could have the illusion of being with fluid dynamics that are coming from Primary Respiration and really be doing very little. We need to understand the spatial relationships of Zone B. This will be covered in all the Phases.

Going too deep, with too much attention/intention, can also overstimulate the Fluid Body. Our attention needs to simply synchronize with Primary Respiration and wait. Let the information come to you as your mind is passive and receptive. The idea that the fluid is deeper than tissue is a misconception that makes for too much focus. This causes the Fluid Body to retreat and fluctuate.

A neutral mind is free to see beyond our usual sensory experience.

We can create a false midline. If the right hand senses the right side and the left hand senses the left side, then we split the fluids in half. Each hand senses the whole Fluid Body.

We can suffocate the breathing of the Fluid Body. Our hands need to be transparent to the incoming tidal forces from outside and the outgoing movements that pass outward through the skin.

Working with energy over-focuses the observer on the bioelectric fields, and the wholeness of fluid becomes laminated.

Do not worry about hurting anyone. Being overly shy can create problems. Just follow easily and let the teaching bring you to a place of balance.

DECOYS

Deception can be obvious or deception can be deeply hidden, so much so that we awaken to find ourselves deceived by our own shadows. It is appropriate to see deception and perhaps not mention it to the patient unless the issue is vital for successful treatment.

Decoys are conscious or subconscious acts by the patient that desynchronize Neutral and turn the fluid in a direction not controlled by Primary Respiration. The direction the fluid takes will not lead to Neutral, as the "will" of the patient is seeking control.

If you notice this happening, rebalance from the feet and wait for Neutral to express itself.

It is difficult to see these decoys because they appear normal.
Look beyond the effects and you will see the cause, easily.

Commonly seen decoys:

- Somatic unwinding
- Patient opens the eyes when the neutral is reached
- Incessant talking
- Clinician talking about personal interests or engaging in conversation with the patient at the expense of the treatment
- The mental following of the treatment by the patient

COMMUNICATION

The teaching of Osteopathy has always included at its core the effort to engage the natural laws of healing. This of course did not mean "laws framed by human hands," as both Still and Sutherland emphasized. Dr. Wales, who led our study group for over thirty years, repeatedly said, "Our goal is to communicate and cooperate with the indwelling laws of healing."

The Fluid Body is a living intelligence that expresses growth and healing through a dynamic state of neutrality. It has a mind that precedes and creates the central nervous system. This means it has an organized Intelligence that creates form, function, and tempo. It is not just a biological fluid that is an effect ... It makes the effect.

Our efforts to communicate with the Fluid Body reveal that the actual pressure of fluid drive is less than one millimeter of mercury. This suggests a remarkable tensionless field that baffles scientific thinking. This low-pressure theory is the result of studying venous pressure in the cranium.

Studies are hard to find, but the intracranial venous pressure is very low (2 mm). When you see a cranial bone and look at the interior surface, you can see the imprint of the venous sinus. This means that the fluid field making the bone is in balance with the low venous pressure. The venous channels are often said to invade the bone. This is misleading. There is no invasion. The venous system and the bone are both made from the same forces, indicating that the pressure in the whole is at a balance point. The system is remarkably poised.

What this means is that if one wishes to listen to the Fluid Body in a child or an adult, then the hands must be in a fluid neutral, thus becoming part of a continuum.

How much pressure does it take to compress a vein on your hand? Try it. It seems very little, yet the venous pressure in the hand is much, much higher than that in the cranium.

This is an interesting topic to explore.

AUTOMATIC SHIFTING

Automatic Shifting is a therapeutic process that was discovered by Dr. Sutherland. Interestingly, it was also described by Dr. Blechschmidt. Blechschmidt called this indwelling capacity for perfect internal synchronization and organization "biokinetics."

Dr. Sutherland's description of this can be found in "The Tour of the Minnow," the last section in *Contributions of Thought*; there is also an article in the 1953 *OCA Journal*.

The process of Automatic Shifting was never taught in courses; apparently, it came about from the skill gained by years of observation. In 1982, after many years of research in my practice, I began to realize the Mind of the Fluid Body was watching my every move. It occurred to me that maybe one could learn how to allow this process to come to the surface in treatment. After several more years, how to engage this process became clear. This is what we are teaching you today. The following conditions permit Automatic Shifting to occur:

1. The patient must have the capacity for Neutral at 2–3 cpm. As you have learned, a CV4 or EV4 may be necessary for this Neutral to express itself. Several treatments may be required for Neutral to emerge easily and naturally for the patient. We never force the fluid or the fluid in the fluid to do anything!
2. The clinician must be able to sense a stillness related to this activity. The particular stillness we engage is the Stillness that resides in the Fluid Body at 2–3 cpm. We call this Second Level Stillness. As one waits in this stillness, Automatic Shifting begins.
3. Automatic Shifting contains many facets:
   a. It moves with precision ... with "uncanny, unerring

potency" that has great accuracy and power. It moves from place to place but disappears between locations ... Where does it go?

b. It prioritizes the lesions ... The healing forces know where to treat ... They are diagnostic. Sutherland points this out (see April 9–12, 1948, in *Contributions of Thought*). This is a map of the patient's needs, drawn by the Tide. In the twenty-five years since I understood this, I have learned a great deal from watching the Master at work ... and it is clear that our diagnostic skills are superseded by this wonderful Mind that displays the treatment.
c. The principle of treatment varies at each point in the Automatic Shifting. As the Tide applies its potency to a particular lesion, the technique is unique and rarely repeated ... As you watch ... think ... feel ... and try to see the styles of treatment ... Let it become your teacher.
d. Eventually the treatment ends ... The fluid goes Still and returns to a new Neutral, one that is deeper and slower than the 2–3 cycles we started with. This is the Long-Tide.
e. The patient rests, and as they do, you draw out the map of what the Tide did.
f. When the patient awakens, show them the map and ask what it means to them ... Often one uncovers history not received earlier.

Try working from the feet to more fully see the Wholeness of the Fluid Body.

AUTOMATIC SHIFTING AND LOCAL FLUID FORCES

Practical

We will work with one extremity to locate the fluid forces at work after the extremity has established a Neutral within itself.

1. Evaluate the extremity, define any strain patterns, and imagine how you might treat it—do not treat.
2. Hold the extremity in a comfortable position for you and become aware of just the fluid forces. Apply a gentle EV4 inside the fluid field and allow the fluid in the whole extremity to come to Neutral.
3. A neutral is when all the fluid in the extremity is breathing as a unit and has a sense of homogenization.
4. Wait in the stillness of the breathing fluid field.
5. Fluid tidal forces will gather and begin to work somewhere within this fluid field.
6. Then these tidal forces will move somewhere else in the extremity or related parts.
7. Notice, are these the places that you were already aware of, as priorities in normalizing the function of the extremity?
8. Keep your mind balanced between the therapeutic effects and the stillness in the whole of the fluid.
9. As the treatment progresses, does it leave the extremity and enter another part of the Fluid Body?
10. The treatment ends. All is quiet. Stillpoint.

11. Did the Tide show you any relationships that were diagnostically useful?
12. This treatment works only if we don't add anything, and only if the neutral can be established successfully.
13. Don't forget to check whether rebalancing is necessary.

THE AUTOMATIC SHIFTING METHOD

W. G. Sutherland often reminds us that the Tide can diagnose and treat. This is a fact. The meaning of this fact will bring us to a completely different understanding of the "magnitude of the heavens of Osteopathy."

Automatic shifting is a self-regulatory, self-potentizing, transmutative process. Our task is to attend to the patient in a precise manner that unveils this process. We can then see the neutral, see the therapeutic process move from place to place, observe its prioritization for the patient's healing as a whole, and end the process in a Stillpoint that fills Zone B.

A simple methodology is as follows:

1. From the feet
2. Synchronize with the breathing in a bowl of water.
3. Sense the whole Fluid Body.
4. Help it to neutral, if necessary.
5. When neutral is established, follow the following:
    a. Place all of your awareness into the stillness of the Fluid Body.
    b. Wait without looking around.
6. The therapeutic forces will gather at a specific site.
7. Observe the therapeutic activity without leaving the stillness.
8. The end point of the treatment is when the therapeutic forces stop and a Stillpoint appears, which merges with the stillness where you are in the Fluid Body.
9. Go to the head and see if rebalancing is required.
10. Draw a diagram of where the therapeutic forces were working and discuss it with the patient.

AUTOMATIC SHIFTING REVIEW

The origin of the term "Automatic Shifting" is from the work of W. G. Sutherland. The basis of this term lies in the repeated observation of self-correcting phenomena within the body. Dr. Sutherland described, quite beautifully, the Automatic Shifting of the central fulcrum at the junction of the straight sinus and the great vein of Galen. This is where the duplication of the dura has its embryological and developmental fulcrum within the central nervous system. Dr. Sutherland said that this fulcrum, within the dural mechanism, was a "suspended automatically shifting still point" through which the potency within the system could be reciprocally maintained. The "Sutherland Fulcrum" is of primordial importance to the health of the body. If it is free to automatically shift, then the neurotrophic functions can operate optimally. However, if Automatic Shifting is restricted, then there will be inhibition of the homeostatic mechanisms and, subsequently, a change throughout the body.

Sutherland also observed this suspended automatically shifting action throughout the body. Within every tissue in the body, regardless of its origin, there is a local, suspended, automatically shifting still point around which the area self-corrects and maintains motion, so that the fluid exchange in the tissue and the neuroendocrine immune function in the extracellular space can be optimally maintained.

To give a very brief description of exactly what kinds of fulcrums we might be thinking about, let us take a look at the beginning of life itself. On the embryonic plate, after the primitive streak appears, the notochord is laid down as the primary line of orientation. It does in fact precede the development of the nervous system by a short period of time and becomes the line of orientation for the geometry of the entire body. The notochord remains in the adult and probably is most clearly appreciated as the center of the nucleus pulposus within the disc—a point, a still point suspended, automatically shifting within a relatively fluid environment. This point remains throughout life and is in fact a shifting fulcrum around which all somato-visceral tissues self-correct. This self-correcting and automatically shifting point is necessary to allow the fluids of life and the integration of the homeostatic mechanisms to maintain themselves at a local level. To be more specific, if we follow the neck of a rib medially, and appreciate the axis that runs through the head and the neck of the rib and project that to the opposite side of the body, we find that both the voluntary and involuntary axes of the rib run directly through this notochordal point. The rib itself and the remaining segmental tissues have an unerring relationship with this point. Every tissue in the body, in fact, has a place that it uses as a point of orientation for its growth and development, through which the potency of the involuntary mechanisms of the body can be delivered into local systems by maintaining a suspended automatically shifting relationship with this point of orientation. When we observe in an air of silence any particular area of the body, we often notice, during the inhalation phase, flexion in the midline with an accommodating external rotation, and during the exhalation phase, midline extension with accommodating internal rotation, all of which is in relation to a local segmental fulcrum. These self-correcting mechanisms in the human body synchronously respond to the silent force of the innate wisdom itself and are under constant scrutiny as a whole unit of a single function, life itself. The homeostatic mechanisms within the body are at work twenty-four hours a day, constantly adapting and automatically shifting so that there is no redundancy, no restriction to the constant, flowing change of life, and under ideal circumstances, the system evolves.

There is something in the human body that, quite profoundly, is always finding, fixing, and then leaving (i.e., automatically shifting). It has few limitations; however, on a physical level, its corrective forces are limited to the hydraulic ability within the system itself and the ability of the central nervous system to inhibit synaptic noise (or facilitation) and project proper efferent information into the extracellular space and recondition the geometry of the tissues and fluid vitality. We are called to assist in this work and allow the system to return from any inertial stresses to Automatic Shifting.

When a patient arrives in our office, he is already under the care of the "Primary Care Physician." When he arrives, he is already being treated. There is a preexisting, prioritized treatment program, and it is part of our job as a member of the team, so to speak, to make an effort to bring into fruition the program of treatment as already outlined by the Primary Care Physician. It is our obligation to sit quietly and observe where in the body the mechanism is at work and, having discovered that, to go directly to the part where the mechanism is working and observe how the mechanism is trying to shift this tissue, and to assist in the process of bringing the area to a point of balance that can be used to shift the tissue back onto its original fulcrum and thus remove its inertial phase.

The mechanism is biphasic. During the inhalation phase, the self-correcting forces in the body are generally trying to establish a state of balanced membranous tension that will then allow, during the exhalation phase, hydraulic forces within the tissues to shift the tissue and fluid to its normal relationship with its embryological and developmental fulcrum. The mechanism uses the inhalation phase for one purpose and the exhalation phase for another. Many times a very small effort on our part to assist the mechanism during the inhalation phase to a point of balanced membranous tension, and then waiting for a change in action during the exhalation phase, makes the difference in allowing the homeostatic mechanisms to operate again.

Many times after doing just a little bit, it is possible to sit back and watch the mechanism automatically shift from one part of the body to another—to bring one part to a state of balanced membranous tension and then use the hydraulic forces within the mechanism to bring about a change in the fulcrums, reduce the inertia, and bring the particular part back in touch with its physiological fulcrum. As we sit quietly and observe this Automatic Shifting, we can learn a great deal about the profound nature of life itself. Many times we work too hard to solve the problem. We give all our attention to the "squeaky wheel" rather than first consulting the concrete prioritized effort of the mechanism. If we sit quietly and are awake to the possibility of this Automatic Shifting, we may observe the Primary Care Physician at work.

The observation is often a diagnostic tool!

I will give you a brief example. A patient comes into the office with a sprained right ankle, and after briefly examining her ankle, I ask her to lie on the table in order to evaluate her comprehensively and to see what kind of strain went through the whole body. Then I place my hands on her system and ask permission to participate. Having done this, I become aware of my own Mechanism. When my own brain and all of its ramblings have surrendered to that moving silence, without any effort it becomes very clear. As that clarity increases, there is only the action of the Mechanism within each of us.

In this particular case, most of the fluid drive and potency within the Mechanism were being delivered for service in the area of the posterior thorax. Observing the Mechanism hard at work in this area, I moved my hands to there to get more in touch with the local fulcrums around which the normal physiological action should take place, and I continued to listen to the Mechanism. I could see that during the inhalation phase it was trying to automatically shift but that it was not possible for it to bring the connective tissue to a state of balanced membranous tension. It seemed to be trying to establish a fluid fulcrum somewhere in the root of the lung on the left side just lateral to the anterior surface of the fourth thoracic vertebra. I tried several times to assist the Mechanism by bringing it to a point of balanced membranous tension around which it would work during the inhalation phase, and then letting it shift during the receding phase. However, the Mechanism continued to work in this area and did not automatically shift to another area. Therefore, after a period of time it occurred to me that there probably was some kind of static process, either metabolic or otherwise, taking place and that the Mechanism was staying in this area because it had not completely transmuted the problem to a point of homeostasis. I took out my stethoscope and listened to the patient's chest. She had a rather dramatic focal wheeze in the middle of the left lung, which was quite obviously pneumonia. She had no symptoms! We gave osteopathic care for the pneumonia and forgot the ankle! She returned in a few days, the pneumonia having resolved. At that point we treated her ankle, and the Mechanism was well and willing to balance the area.

The point is that the patient's Mechanism had prioritized the needs of the patient, and it is our effort to cooperate with the prioritization as it expresses itself within the patient. In this particular case, which is really not uncommon, the Mechanism was working in an area that seemed unrelated to the patient's chief complaint; however, the Mechanism was working in this area because the "Primary Care Physician" had already determined that the patient had pneumonia and was hard at work taking care of her before we arrived on the scene. I think we have all had this experience of treating a patient for one thing and having something else get better, and this clearly demonstrates the principles of Automatic Shifting and prioritization within the Mechanism. If we can learn to cooperate with it, to follow it and use it as a diagnostic tool, we will probably find that the Mechanism is not only intelligent but very compassionate and very much interested in the whole life of the individual. We as physicians must be patient, and, having done this, perhaps will be able to dig deeper into the beauty of life itself.

For me personally, the observation of Automatic Shifting is becoming a tremendous diagnostic tool and is simultaneously yielding a deep appreciation of the Stillness that always seems to end every treatment.

CHILDREN'S OBSERVATIONS

In 1979, a dance teacher from New York, who summered in rural Maine, told me that during her treatments she could feel the warm fluid movements. This occurred on a regular basis after she had her first three treatments. She was a professional dancer. In the summer, she taught children to dance and express fluidity in motion. She said she wondered if children could naturally feel what we called Primary Respiration.

Children seven to nine years old were asked to observe their mind and report what they saw with their imagination.

Imagination: to picture to oneself something not present to the original five senses. It is used here to acknowledge imagination as a creative act of the highest degree of insight.

As the children observed their inner world, this is what they reported:

1. It felt like a sea of many people that were fighting over me. (Joana, grade 3)
2. My imagination works with the whole body and looks like crawling on grass. (Jason, grade 4)
3. Mine looks like a brain, feels like a big circle in my head. (JoAnn, grade 2)
4. My imagination is like a blob. It changes shape, size, and color. If you could feel it, it would feel slippery and spongy. It scoops up ideas and squeezes them into one idea. It fixes it up so that it is as good as can be and sends it to my mind. My mind sends it to my hand and I do it. (Alon, grade 4)
5. It felt like someone was in a boat. It felt like I was in a boat. (Daniel, grade 3)
6. My imagination changes by the minute; now it's in my

stomach. (Jacob, grade 2)

7. Opening and closing. (Ryan, grade 2)
8. My wind has many thoughts. Today her thought is a bird. Not just any bird though! (Erin, grade 4)
9. Blue fire, fierce fire. (Daniel, grade 4)
10. I can't go inside my mind without going side to side. It's so windy. I find out that the wind is wavy, and it has special vitamins to pick up things. (Renee, grade 3)
11. If it is trapped, it feels like it is going to die. (Amy, grade 4)
12. Wee-hee-hee-hee-hee-hee. (Keith, grade 4)
13. It wants to be free. It doesn't want to be in an enclosed area. It likes to just be a nice summer breeze. (Jennifer, grade 4)
14. Freedom! (Nicholas, grade 4)
15. Very, very wavy. (Angela, grade 4)

Instinct is present throughout our lives; it knows. The skill we seek is innate.

A CHRISTMAS GREETING FROM ANNE WALES

1997

On Earth Peace,

Good Will Toward Men

Dear Jim,

Christmas Greetings and Best Wishes for 1997. I was glad to hear from you and of you. It has been a busier year than seems probable, but at last I am writing to you. I am glad Will's picture got to you. That does show his spirit. How everything going in this living human body influences everything else!

In my last conversation with Will (spring 1954) I asked him what accounts for the fluctuation of the C.S.F. in its natural cavity and he said he didn't know. He did teach that both it and the motility of the C.N.S. shifted the Automatic Shifting Fulcrum of the RTM which moves the cranial bones at the sutures to provide the change of shape for the brain as a living organ. I can't seem to hold the three dimensional picture together in one piece, but I try.

I have told Pietro that he can come to visit.

Love, Anne

It's the not-yet in the now,

the taste of the fruit that does not-yet exist,

hanging the blossom on the bough.

–Laurens van der Post, *Venture to the Interior*, Harcourt, 1979

SYNCHRONIZATION

Synchronization with Primary Respiration is "being with the Health."

This is always our first step, if we wish to work with the slower rates (less than 8–14 per minute) and the intention of the Tide.

As one works with synchronization, this unlocks the perception to more subtle and powerful landscapes and exposes the slower rates to our observer. This allows one to begin to "see" how to cooperate with the natural laws and, as many of our teachers have stated, is the foundation of Osteopathy.

As we discipline ourselves to work with synchronization, clarity and transparency in the Mechanism will naturally unfold… making our diagnostics more keen and allowing us to see the therapeutic forces rather than the "effects"…

FLUID LANGUAGE

2–3 cpm
Dynamic Stillness
Stillpoint
Breath of Life
Potency
Long-Tide
Spiritual Fulcrum
Henson's Node
Midline
The Spark
Ignition
The Tide
The Potency
Hammering
Life Forces
Soft
Vectorial
Fluid Body
Fluid in the Fluid
Axial Fluctuations
Fluid Fluctuations
Whole
Fluid Drive
Fluid Fulcrum
Balanced Fluid Tension
Balance Point
Soul

Biokinetics
Automatic Shifting
Neurotrophic Flow
Trophicity
Metabolic Fluid
Field
Original Blueprint
Health
Imago Dei
Groundswell
Molding
Transmutation
Rate 6/10
False Fulcrums
Tempo
Fluency
Hydraulic Leverage
Disengagement
Heat
Lamination
Rebalancing
Therapeutic Phase
Inhalation Phase
Exhalation Phase
Stillpoint
Biodynamic
Silence

Fluid Hydraulics
Position, Form, Space
Neutral

Stillness
Balance Point
Pause

Language, to be precise, must be as absolute as a mathematical proof.

It must contain the perfect, the imaginary, and the infinite.

PHASE TWO UPDATE

The Mind of the Fluid Body creates the central nervous system.

We learn that we cannot control the Fluid Body ... We can lesion it with our intentions, but we can rebalance the patient whenever required. This keeps our work safe.

We are learning communication with a Higher Mind. As we adjust to not using our own personal forces to treat, and to not relating to lesions, our senses are converted to a new landscape ... then things become much easier.

We also discover, in discussion with others, that there is a general consensus on when the patient is at Neutral. We begin to appreciate common truths around which the profession has long survived.

During the second practical, we sense the wholeness of Zone A and the wholeness of Zone B. From the Central Stillness, Zone A extends to the edge of the skin. The tone of A feels like somatic tension. We try to feel this as a unit along with the Central Stillness. Zone B is very different. It expresses itself from the Central Stillness to a boundary not determined by the skin; it may feel like it is either around or within Zone A. Its tone is protoplasmic, ranging from stiff to fluently soft. We attempt to find the interface between A and B. We rebalance the Fluid Body as a whole through the fulcrum of the Central Stillness (rather than above and below the foramen magnum, as we did in Phase One).

Let's review some of the history of this curriculum ... the teachers and the mentors, the story of long relationships with highly skilled American Osteopaths who chose "the road less traveled." Biodynamics is not "my" teaching. It is the continuum of a legacy passed to me by mentors who spent their personal time, energy, and resources in their teaching to me. This particular teaching was not undertaken within structured courses (although I have also completed more than 8,000 hours of postgraduate courses). All my mentors were in general practice, not manipulative medicine, as many are today.

My first actual cranial course was in 1966 at Kirksville College of Osteopathic Medicine ... it was not for students, but another student and I cut classes to go and were welcomed to join the ten or so physicians taking the course. It was hard! When one of our clinical teachers found out we were skipping class for a cranial course, he gave an unannounced test. We were absent, so we flunked the test. The zero on the test dropped our average so low that we had to outline the entire course textbook to gratify the professor.

Right from the first course, there were people who reflected the cranial work but some who really supported it. My most intimate mentors were these:

George Laughlin, D.O. (A. T. Still's grandson and avid supporter of WGS)

John Chace, D.O. (Ob-gyn who treated babies when the head presented during delivery... he was very skilled and supported WGS)

Irvin (Kim) Korr, Ph.D. (Professor of Physiology ... author of many articles on the Osteopathic lesion ... an avid fan of cranial work)

Keith Buzzell, D.O. (head of the Department of Osteopathic Medicine and coauthor of *The Physiological Basis of Osteopathic Medicine*)

I saw all these men on a regular basis as I studied at Kirksville for my doctorate.

In 1966 I was awarded a predoctoral fellowship in anatomy and Osteopathic method. My mentor for the five years of that program was George Snyder, Ph.D., professor of anatomy and embryology. He was an Osteopathic thinker who taught us Osteopathic embryology and wrote at length on "the embryological development of the fascia."

He was a perfectionist and a great teacher. I did 150 dissections and lectures under his care.

After Kirksville, I mentored with Ruby Day, DO. She studied and then taught with WGS from 1936 to 1953. She refused to follow the mechanical model of Magoun, and consequently she left teaching with him and the Sutherland Cranial Teaching Foundation in 1953. I worked with her from 1973 to 1986. She died soon after.

In 1978, Stefan Hagopian, DO and I asked Anne Wales to start a closed study group. She was barely able to walk, but she still said yes, and subsequently she became restored in the company of her new "children." She continued to teach us until her death. My last day with her was in 2006 ... a long and loving friendship.

In 1978, I met Dr. Rollin Becker. He was very kind to me over the next ten years. In 1982, I introduced biodynamics in a lecture ... The audience thought I was crazy. As they confronted me, Dr. Becker stepped into the chaos and said, "Leave him alone, he knows what he is saying" ... I was terrified. Over the next few days as I lectured, he stood near me and intervened when all the mechanical osteopaths became upset. He taught me about love and speaking only from my love for this work. He mentored me and was my personal trainer when I joined the Sutherland Cranial Teaching Foundation that year.

From 1978 to 1993, I either took or taught a total of 125 courses with the Sutherland Cranial Teaching Foundation. There are many stories here. Dr. Becker really opened the door to Neutral as a starting point of treatment.

Many retiring DOs have sent me their cranial papers and skulls, because they wanted to support this lineage: Tom Schooley, Ruby Day (via Steven Kissel), Anna Biddle, Drs. Barnes and Hull (the personal secretaries and caregivers to WGS in his last years at his home in California. His home was called "the fulcrum," where he could see the lighthouse over the Pacific Ocean that he loved so much). Alan Becker, DO, also mentored me. We exchanged audiotapes with comments and discussion about the Fluid Body. He was a great teacher. He brought his brother to WGS ... and left teaching when the politics got more important than the Tide. He was planning to audit the courses just before he died because, as he said, "I Love Osteopathy." He was in his mid-eighties ... as was Jacques Duval, DO, of Paris, who studied Biodynamics with a razor-sharp eye until his death. He had a great capacity to love, and I truly miss his dear friendship ... There is a lot more ... but this should begin to meet the request for a list of my mentors ...

So ... back to the present.

As a practical, we can draw pictures of Zone A, Zone B, and the things we feel ... then we can clarify each drawing and make a list of our findings, and develop our language.

BIODYNAMICS: WHAT DOES IT MEAN?

The word "Biodynamic" was chosen for these courses because of the parallels discovered between the work of W. G. Sutherland, DO, and Erich Blechschmidt, MD. The word was positioned in medicine by Dr. Blechschmidt, and, as you will see, we have extended it to envelop the fluid dynamics of Primary Respiration expressed by William Sutherland, DO.

Even though embryology is at the very roots of Osteopathy, no one to my knowledge has seen the similarities between the observations of Dr. Blechschmidt and Dr. Sutherland as regards the indwelling fluid activity of creation and healing extending not just in utero but throughout life.

The word "biodynamic" has a special meaning when seen from the summation of both men's efforts to unveil the movements of Life. Both men are recognized as pioneers. Both men, one working with growth and development and the other working with healing through transmutation, described similar processes in the internal activity of protoplasmic fields. When I saw the similarities I was elated and doubtful, as it seemed almost unimaginable, but as I studied further the parallels were everywhere, unavoidable, and precise. The improvement in clinical outcomes was amazing.

The foundations of Osteopathy are in embryology. This has been forgotten by all but a few Osteopaths. The embryological segment has become replaced by the vertebral segment. Most Osteopaths are thinking about bony lesions and direct action to relieve "nerve pressure" as the basis of treatment rather than a direct awareness of the indwelling capacity of natural laws to express themselves in a symphony of therapeutic movements.

The role of the autonomic nervous system in disease as a principle based in embryology is being neglected in our thinking and educational orientation. The segmentation of the embryo is the foundation of how we think, even biomechanically. Our elders all thought from these principles as they tried to "excite or inhibit" functions of the autonomics.

Osteopathy is an applied art.

Will Sutherland was interested in embryology. He encouraged his students to read embryology. He used embryology as the foundation of his work on the extremities (see "Power Points" in Phase Six). He was grounded in a working knowledge of embryology, as you shall see in this and other commentaries.

My first exposure to embryology was in Kirksville (1965) ... I was spiritually awed by the unfolding process and the Mind behind all this beauty of growth and development.

My anatomy fellowship mentor, Dr. George Snyder, wrote papers on the embryological development of the fascia. We studied embryology and segmentation in order to be more effective at diagnosis and treatment. At the time, Pottinger was the text that we depended on the most, but in recent times the works of Michael Kuchera, DO, have better served our purposes.

Later, in 1980, John Harakal, DO, then the president of the Sutherland Cranial Teaching Foundation in the US, asked me to do a lecture on the development of the central nervous system for the foundation's basic course.

As I set forth to review and update my knowledge of the subject, I first went to Dr. Sutherland's writings, reading and rereading "The Tour of the Minnow."

As usual, when one reviews the masters in any tradition, it feels like a first reading ... One truly wonders if one ever read it before.

As I read, I ran across the term "lamina terminalis" ... I did not know what it was ... so ... I tried to look it up ... not easily forthcoming ... book after book on anatomy was naked on the topic ... One embryology text showed a picture of lamina terminalis as the membrane closing the anterior neuropore of the third ventricle. It was obvious that the lamina terminalis was not common knowledge.

How did Sutherland know this? I do not know, but I suspect he was patient in his observations of involuntary motion ... a task that most DOs would find uninteresting and tedious. He watched without overlaying his ideas; remember, he was the first to see Primary Respiration in a medical context ... And he had nothing to lead him.

Sutherland was an *Osteopathic* thinker and explorer.

He discovered what science cannot, as yet, find ... a pattern of motion in the patient that could be appreciated in both diagnosis and treatment, leading his profession into new territory. The motion had a rhythm; he called it Primary Respiration because it was different from Thoracic Respiration and seemed to be more essential to life.

At first, I thought that the lamina terminalis was just the name of a place, but Sutherland points to it as a place to and from which the central nervous system takes its motion. As a fulcrum. It is a functional pivot and a doorway to the "sea around us."

As I was totally frustrated with the information in the books, I turned to the librarian at the University of New England College of Osteopathic Medicine where I was an off-campus clinical professor of Osteopathic family practice.

After thousands of dollars and months of waiting, thirty or forty articles from all over the world that contained the words "lamina terminalis" arrived in the mail ... Most were vague, but one article mentioned that the lamina terminalis was the point where the torus opticus unfolded into a myriad of functions in the central nervous system's development (see central nervous system lecture, Phase One). I was aghast.

Sutherland clearly saw the importance of the lamina terminalis as a "fulcrum" for the pattern and power of central nervous system motion, and now we find that his kernel of truth was pregnant. The lamina terminalis was a fulcrum for the growth and development of the central nervous system as well as many other functions (see Phases Three through Six). The story of his clear understanding will come through as we proceed in this commentary.

Will saw the importance of the lamina terminalis and somehow he knew of its function in the unfolding of life before the science of embryology discovered it.

My first lecture was, for me, exciting news about the wisdom of what Sutherland noticed and how deep this truth was.

Unfortunately, not everyone thought I was brilliant. Some of the board members were certain that I was crazy. There was panic and doubt all directed at me in a flurry of rejection ... But four physicians stepped into the fire with me and supported what I had found in my reading: Rollin Becker, Robert Fulford, John Harakal, and Jacques Duval ... They literally called off the irritated mass of experts.

I was confused at the frantic response. Some faculty members were so angry at me that they thought I invented the whole thing ... which of course I did not ... I was following Will's words to the letter. Most of that lecture is in Phase One.

My interest did not wane. I read and read ... all kinds of strange (to me) articles ... I was seeing, however slowly, the deep connection between the Health as Still taught, Primary Respiration as Sutherland described it, and the fluids and the forces of creation that unfold our inner embryonic world, as Blechschmidt described them.

In another five years I was a real "nut case" ... often dreaming that my embryo was talking to me ... I fell in love with the livingness and sweet silence in which all unfolding occurs.

My critics were hard; they clung to the safety of the past and their position as teachers ... I was forty years old. They were twenty years older. Now I am sixty-five and can understand the critics better ... something Will was confronted with. Most critics are cowards, never directly debating the issues, only commenting in dark corners. The critics have helped me look deeper and harder and have been most helpful in my developing these connections. They have my gratitude for pushing me into clear water.

"A little learning is a dangerous thing; drink deep, or taste not the Pierian spring" ... this quote is from a poem by Alexander Pope entitled "An Essay on Criticism" and was set in the title page of the first edition of Will's book. The poem is very useful, as it gives insight into the constant rejection Will digested in his easy manner and kindness ... He is a role model one can easily admire for his tolerance and neutrality.

I know I have not said what the use of the term "biodynamic" means ... but I am getting there ... the story goes on ...!

As my research into embryology continued, I was directed to Blechschmidt's "A Symposium on the Development of the Basicranium" by my childhood neighbor, Frank Willard, Ph.D. All along the way he has been a good critic and generously answered questions as they arose ...

I realized I was "out on a limb" ... alone.

I discovered descriptions in embryology that paralleled Sutherland's comments about his observations gleaned from listening to the fluids as they responded to Primary Respiration. These parallels narrowed and met ...

There are pictures of the metabolic fields in Blechschmidt's writings, in particular near the end of the text *Biokinetics and Biodynamics of Human Differentiation* ... These pictures describe forces at work in the metabolic fields ... well ... They are the same as what Sutherland described. The pictures in Magoun's text are exactly the same (pages 100 and 101, third edition).

For example, in one of Blechschmidt's figures there are two men inside the fluid field facing each other and pushing toward each other

... In other words, the two men are bringing the metabolic field toward the "center" ... the same as in a CV4 where the forces of the fluid in the fluid are brought to a central point, creating Neutral ... through which therapeutics become active.

Another picture in Blechschmidt clearly defines a spreading apart of the metabolic field that replicates Sutherland's base spread done with only the gentlest of touch ... This has been called EV4 in the Biodynamic Model because the Direction of Ease in the fluid field is the opposite of that in a CV4. Other pictures represent what we would call disengagement and opposing physiological activity.

As I saw all this, the light came on ... Both of the men, one with a microscope and one with his hands, were watching the same process. It seemed too simple to be true, but there it was. I was a little overwhelmed ... everything stopped ... the partitions came down. The oneness was incomprehensible ... The models of Primary Respiration I had been taught and used for years shattered and a "breath of something other" entered the shoreline of my little mind.

Intuitively I felt a warmth and admiration for Still and Sutherland ... also, I saw again how long it takes to be aware of nature's laws at work in patients, rather than adding laws "framed by human hands." I grew up in that moment ... no more compromise.

Sutherland's perceptual journey was critical for his understanding. He had to change how he worked and how he thought ... The perceptual reclothing of his awareness was a hard task. He had to rethink his formulations over and over ...

Because of this synthesis, I reread and cataloged all of the perceptual steps I could recognize in the complete text of *Contributions of Thought*. The key was the observer changing ... and ... being free of bias.

What is the word "Biodynamic" all about ...?

The premise of indwelling therapeutic forces inside of us came through Still and Sutherland very clearly ... so clearly that many have decided that it is just philosophy.

Sutherland followed Still almost word for word. My whole entry into Osteopathy was because I trusted nature more than politicians or businessmen ... When I read Still, I was sold ... Then I applied to Kirksville, announcing to them in my application that I was only applying to one school and if rejected I would stay in graduate school until they accepted me ... Now some twenty years later there I was, immersed in a sea of truth from many sources ... I was elated ... but there was more.

Sutherland's model of Primary Respiration was "a house under the sea" with all the doors and windows open and the Tide moving through with ease, bringing form, function, and healing.

Blechschmidt's sense of the metabolic fields in embryos was that they were biodynamic; that is, they were an expression of an outside, extra-genetic force of creation, known only to the embryo ... not scientists, but the embryo ... an Ocean that is through us, creating involuntary motions (biokinetics) and self-correcting activities (Automatic Shifting).

An Ocean. A House. Transparency of the Whole to the creative forces.

As I assimilated these little pieces, years passed into the early nineties ... but there is more to the question. What is biodynamics and what is behind the word!

Metabolic fields, whether in embryos or adults, are about the death of the old and the building of the new ...

Metabolic ... catabolic ... anabolic ... in this metabolic fire, what is it that synchronizes the death and growth of form and function? What creates the death and what transmits the boundary of the function that is unfolding?

Metabolism does not happen without a catalyst, and at the most essential level that catalyst is unknown ... Sutherland used an ancient Greek word to describe the metabolic shift ...

Transmutation (see Ovid's *Metamorphoses,*) ... a complete change ... a change so dramatic that it was akin to a change in species, not genus ... the change is a result of transmutation.

Blechschmidt did not have the tools to go as far as Sutherland in this direction.

Sutherland's hands became transparent to this truth. He himself grew into an intimate relationship with the biodynamic sea around us, to the point where he saw through the effects into another fulcrum (cause) ... that could only be called that which lies beyond transmutation ... the Breath of Life ... herein is the Power of Creation entering the Sea, which has the Potency to transmute biostasis, the enemy of growth and healing, and reestablish freshness.

These facts may seem poetic, but the facts stand by themselves, unalterable, precise, and unerring. A Mystery known only to the innocence that an embryo images to us, but a concrete fact.

As the Biodynamic Model and methodology grew from 1978 to the mid-1990s, many people became interested again in embryology and began to study the unfoldment of life.

I caution the reader to remember that Sutherland went beyond the form into the cause that makes embryology happen ... This is a different study from that of embryological milestones.

Biodynamics is not about forms or formats ... it is about the intimate manifestations of Primary Respiration as a creative and therapeutic force that transmutes the old and carries the image of the new into place.

This ability to transmute lies behind all success in treatment; behind all spatial and temporal interfaces that unfold as development and growth occur ... through neutral homeostasis.

The "Sea Around Us" is Biodynamic.

As yet, embryology has not caught up with Sutherland—or Still, for that matter ...

I do not encourage the study of embryology beyond a point of basic understanding and awe.

Rather, study Primary Respiration ... Look behind the effects ... What is cause ... and what are the means of communication with that cause and its intention?

The test of these truths is not in logic but in the clinical advantage they bring to the varieties of suffering a country doctor witnesses ... All patients benefit in many ways from hands that diagnose and treat from these foundations ...

Still called it Life, "that slow vivifying force coming forth from God." Sutherland called it Primary Respiration ... It is One.

Biodynamics means all of this and more ...

Blechschmidt chose the word to make the point that there was an extra-genetic force at work in the creation and the unfolding of embryonic life.

Sutherland saw that force at work as transmutation, coming from the Sea Around Us ... and ultimately from the Creator.

Mix the paints of these two men and you will find the word "biodynamic" and its meaning.

RECOMMENDED READING

Sutherland, W. G., *Contributions of Thought,* The Cranial Academy, 1967.

Sutherland, W. G., *Teachings in the Science of Osteopathy,* Rudra Press, 1990.

Magoun, H., *Osteopathy in the Cranial Field,* First Edition, The Cranial Academy, 1997.

Blechschmidt, E., *The Beginnings of Human Life,* Springer, 1977.

Blechschmidt, E., and Gasser, R., *Biokinetics and Biodynamics of Human Differentiation,* North Atlantic Books, 2012.

Blechschmidt, E., *The Ontogenetic Basis of Human Anatomy,* North Atlantic Books, 2004.

DeHaan, R. L., *Organogenesis,* Holt, Rinehart and Winston, 1965.

Opitz, J. M., "The Developmental Field Concept in Clinical Genetics," *The Journal of Pediatrics 101,* no. 5 (1982): 805-809.

Seifriz, W., *Seifriz on Protoplasm,* a video available on YouTube.

Pischinger, A., *The Extracellular Matrix and Ground Regulation,* North Atlantic Books, 2007.

REFERENCE TO PALPATION OF THE EMBRYO

In his book *The Beginnings of Human Life* (1977), Dr. Erich Blechschmidt writes:

> The bicellular stage is the most elementary and primitive cellular system of the organism. Its two cells are substantially interconnected by a submicroscopically narrow gap. It is the first site of an intercellular particle exchange, and by means of these molecular movements (local metabolic movements), which may be postulated on the basis of the permeability of the cell's limiting membranes, the two blastomeres cling to each other in a sort of suction process. The forces holding the cells together can be demonstrated experimentally by attempting to separate them artificially; indeed, the forces can even be sensed by the touch of a finger. ... In vivo, these forces are certainly upheld by metabolic functions, and not simply by mechanical and purely physical forces. The latter do not exist in the living being, as shown by numerous observations. The attempt to apply a purely formal (rationalistic), or a purely mechanical (mechanistic), or a purely chemical (materialistic), mode of reasoning in human embryology would mean to confound in a gross manner the technique of study with the object to be studied.

Blechschmidt, *The Beginnings of Human Life*, Springer, 1977.

THE FUNCTIONS OF THE FLUID BODY

Practical

If we can successfully discriminate between the various motions related to Fluid Body dynamics, we can set our mind at ease in our understanding of what these motions represent and what they mean. This practical session is purely observational, except for the rebalancing at the end of the session.

Synchronize with the Health and maintain a vital connection with its presence throughout the entire observational exercise. This prevents lesioning the patient and also provides communication with the consciousness of the Fluid Body, which lets it open and reveal its intentions.

All the functions of the Fluid Body, as we are now describing them, occur at a tempo of two to three cycles per minute. If the rate changes, then detailed observation of the functions we have discussed is not possible. If for any reason you are not sure or are unclear, check with someone who has knowledge and experience..

The goal of this session is to have a clear observation of a variety of functions.

FLUID BODY LESIONS

Practical

Before we transition to doing a CV4 or EV4, we need to look at the state of the Fluid Body, which generally is in lesion. It is very easy to think that a fluid lesion is a therapeutic wave and follow it to an end point. All this does is cause more compensation. But because the Fluid Body goes into a pause, people often think that they are at a dynamic stillpoint.

Make a list of your findings relative to the patterns in the Fluid Body. Try to use the information that we have discussed so far. The following are some things you might notice:

1. Rate
2. Fluid Body Motion Zone A
3. Fluid Body Motion Zone B
4. Longitudinal Fluctuation
5. Lateral Fluctuation
6. Fluid Drive
7. Where's the Fulcrum for:
    a. The Lesion
    b. The Whole Fluid Body
    c. The Stillness of the Fluid Body

"Do you see the point?"

W. G. Sutherland, D.O.

REFERENCES TO "IDLING" IN *CONTRIBUTIONS OF THOUGHT*

Recommended reading: *Contributions of Thought* by William Garner Sutherland. Here are a few brief quotes, with dates, where he mentions idling:

Cerebrospinal Fluid Fluctuation and Central Nervous System Motility – April 9, 1948

"Bring the fluctuation of the cerebrospinal fluid down to a brief idling in its fluctuation ... That is what we are trying to do when we say "compress the bulb."

When you reach the idling period, you will detect an immediate change ... Not only in the hands, the extremities, but all through the viscera, the connective tissue and the fascia. An interchange that occurs between all the fluids of the body."

Techniques for Incitation and Repression of Cerebrospinal Fluid Fluctuation – April 10, 1948

"We are bringing the fluctuation down to the desired point, that brief rhythmic period of fluctuation of the body of the cerebrospinal fluid. ... It is what we want to get in "compression of the bulb." ... bring the fluctuation to a central point in vibration, the motor is idling, and the interchange between all the fluids of the body occurs."

Diagnosis and Treatment Using the Tide – April 12, 1948

"I want you to see the whole tide coming to what we call the 'balance' as balance between two scales. That is the point where the mechanism is idling, neither ebbing out or flowing in, but right on the neutral point. That is why we say "rhythmic balance interchange."

LONGITUDINAL FLUCTUATION

When you visualize the pattern of the longitudinal fluctuation of the cerebrospinal fluid, as you have experienced it in your palpation in the past, what do you come to?

The longitudinal fluctuation begins at the coccyx at the beginning of the inhalation phase, ascends to the core-link and enters the foramen magnum at the mid-inhalation phase, flows forward, filling the posterior, middle, and anterior cranial fossa with its potency, and ends. During exhalation it has a pattern of fluctuation that descends from the ethmoid region to the coccyx, completing its elliptical pathway at the end of the exhalation phase.

The reciprocal tensions in the fluids of the body carry an organized pattern of potency, which is the Breath of Life building and maintaining the architecture of the body. These reciprocal tensions of potency within the fluid create reciprocal tension layers that then guide the cellular arrangement of the tissues, during both development and adult life. One place where this is easily seen is in the development of the meninges, where there is a layering of the mesenchyme into the pia, arachnoid, and dura. As potency enters fluid, it patterns the fluid, and as a result the fluid has an inherent reciprocal tension. This reciprocal tension of the fluid is manifest as a hydraulic force, a noncompressible quality that is balanced with the atmospheric pressure and as a living biomolecular, biochemical continuum.

Having established some of the fundamental principles that reflect the inherent qualities of the normal patterning, let us now review some irregularities in the pattern of the longitudinal fluctuation.

Before discussing techniques for correction, it is necessary to review the basic physiology that dictates these techniques. The reciprocal tension membrane, its pattern and shape, must be understood. The tentorium cerebelli is a pyramid-shaped structure; the base of the pyramid widens during the inhalation phase so that the angulation between the sides of the tentorium becomes more obtuse. During exhalation it becomes narrower at the base, and angles are more acute. Dr. Sutherland discovered that if this reciprocal tension membrane is held in a position of exhalation, then eventually the entire system, including the inherent motility of the central nervous system and the fluctuation of the cerebrospinal fluid, will align itself with the pattern that the operator is introducing into the mechanism. Dr. Sutherland observed that if he held the occipital area in extension, the mechanism would slowly quiet down to a full exhalation and still point and then would start up again; during this process there would be an exchange within the body on many levels of physiology that stimulated the immune system, the lymphatic system, the nervous system ... in fact, quite profoundly influenced the whole physiology. A technique that he called the CV4 was designed to stimulate and to repattern the physiology of the body. Dr. Sutherland also discovered that in placing the mechanism into its inhalation pattern, that is, influencing the bones and membranes so that the tent becomes more flattened, eventually the system will take itself down to a still point and a kind of Neutral will be felt in the fluid with a repatterning of some of the irregularities in the cerebrospinal fluid. We most commonly hear about this type of technique in terms of resuscitation of patients that have lost their heartbeat and respiration, and so the mechanism has to be pumped up again, so to speak, by rocking the temporal bones and in some cases holding the temporal bones in external rotation. However, the principle of trying to resuscitate this mechanism, by taking it into a position of external rotation and influencing the mechanism in that direction and then taking it back to internal rotation, is aimed at stimulating the longitudinal fluctuation of the cerebrospinal fluid by this alternating flexion and extension. These resuscitation techniques that he described were for reestablishing the Breath of Life.

There is one technique which is extremely useful and more comfortable under ordinary conditions of general practice. As described earlier, there are different kinds of irregularities in the longitudinal fluctuation of the cerebrospinal fluid; these can be diagnostic. This particular technique allows an easier diagnostic view. It opens the mechanism very slowly and allows the physician to stay in the diagnostic mode throughout the procedure. This is extremely useful in assessing how well the longitudinal fluctuation of the cerebrospinal fluid can recover from an irregularity in its patterning. It also is useful in assessing the amount of inertia in that irregularity. We are able to find out how easily the mechanism will be able to correct itself, and, diagnostically, that can give us a sense of how deeply this irregularity in the fluctuation of the cerebrospinal fluid may be imbedded in the physiology of the patient. Some patients will respond quite quickly and others will respond slowly. Each individual's ability to adapt to stress modalities is different. A diagnosis is a very individualized event. As clinicians, we must know how easy it is going to be to get this system to return to normal. Using these techniques and staying in a diagnostic mental framework can be extremely useful in terms of knowing at what level we might want to enter into communication with the patient, and also what level of additional support the patient might need depending upon how much resistance we see in the system. This technique is one that very gently and slowly takes the system into its inhalation mode so that we will be influencing the osseous and membranous structure to go into an inhalation pattern. We do this very gently and synchronously so that we can monitor the quality of response in the system and the ease with which that system is able to reregulate itself. On the other hand, if we try to force these changes into the physiology, it will not give the central nervous system time to adjust to the influences and we may end up getting an emotional release in the patient that is not therapeutic.

This technique basically involves placing the two fifth fingers together in the midline under the occiput just below the union and taking the occipital bone into a slight amount of flexion—I would say trying to just influence the occipital bone into flexion until we feel a very, very slight change in the fluid, and then wait. During the time that we are waiting we will keep our observation on the tongue-and-groove articulation between the basiocciput and the occipital bone and the temporal bone. We will then increase the transverse diameter across the lateral angles of the occipital bones (which is the opposite movement from what we do in a CV4) so that we are actually opening the transverse diameter across lateral angles and out through the asterion, thus flattening the tent and stimulating the inhalation phase of the primary respiratory mechanism. Having encouraged this increase in the transverse diameter, we will start to feel a give in the temporal bones, at which time we can gently lift our forces forward through the occipital bone toward the metopic suture, which will result in a slight external rotation of the temporal bones and allow the system to adjust and engage its entire physiology so that eventually we get this nice neutral feeling in all the tissues through the entire mechanism, including the fluid, and we come to a still point. Following, we see a repatterning of the longitudinal fluctuation. If this does not occur, it represents a seriously unyielding problem. How easily the longitudinal fluctuation in the cerebrospinal fluid repatterns is diagnostic. We continue to make observations after the still point for three phases of inhalation to get some idea of how the patterning in that longitudinal fluctuation is going to change or is not going to change, and then, of course, a follow-up visit becomes imperative because we need to see whether or not this change is sustained over a period of time. Frequently there may not be much of a change in the longitudinal fluctuation at the time of treatment, but when the patient returns, a change is obvious. It remains a topic of amazement to me how gentle and subliminal the intelligent wisdom of this mechanism is. It can bring the patient into balance within a time frame that is acceptable to the entire nervous system in terms of a change in the psyche and the soma. It is our job as clinicians to follow that wisdom and to use our communication with that wisdom as a diagnostic tool so that we get the feel of what this mechanism is trying to tell us about the quality of change in this patient. However, we also have to be aware of the fact that in some cases things do not change because we have not applied the technique properly or we have used a technique therapeutically when it should have been used diagnostically. It is important for the clinician not to have any expectations therapeutically about the effect of a specific technique until he has taken it through its diagnostic phase, be that brief or longer, so that he knows whether or not this technique has been therapeutic or whether or not it has been diagnostic. It is very important to keep this in one's mind at all times. If the technique does not work, it does not mean that there is something wrong with the patient, nor does it mean that there is anything wrong with our observation, but it does mean that we have to look at this patient longer and more deeply and look for other keys that will help us know where to place our influences in such a direction that we can reintegrate the patient into a functional unit.

From this discussion one can see that understanding the anatomy and the physiology of the system is absolutely imperative in using the techniques and that if we do not understand exactly what these techniques are designed to do, applying them is not going to be of much use to us diagnostically.

Man is triune. He has a body, a soul, and a mind. People do not feel a sense of well-being unless these three aspects function as a unit, unpartitioned! The longitudinal fluctuation is intimately connected with the perceptual fields and sensory experience of the Soul. A pattern of irregularity can severely limit one's sense of security, safety, and Love.

FLUID ACTIVITIES

1. Two and a half cycles per minute is primarily a fluid wave.
2. This is an internal motion within all bodily fluids.
3. It fluctuates and cycles.
4. It can automatically shift its therapeutic leverage from one site to another.
5. It has fulcrums for self-regulation.
6. It generates fulcrums for self-correcting events.
7. The Potency of the Tide inside the fluid is an effect of the Breath of Life, but is not the Breath of Life itself. This is important.
8. Fluids are internally decisive in embryonic development and the healing process.
9. In longitudinal fluctuation (inhalation phase) the Tidal intentions can be appreciated.
10. The dominant rate at death is two and a half cycles per minute, slowly yielding to the Long-Tide.
11. Fluid forces do not recognize rational boundaries between structure and function; it is *form*.

EMBRYOLOGICAL SEEDS

1. Our explorations and interest should not be limited by models.
2. Embryogenesis is not modulated by the central nervous system. Forces inside fluids make decisions.
3. The "self" of the immune system appears before the central nervous system and before "non-self" is created.
4. We are searching for Health; we are attempting to follow its direction moment to moment as it consciously creates living motion toward perfection.
5. Health is the emergence of the Original, creative genius of life, not a result of man-made remedies.
6. The forces of embryogenesis become the forces of healing in the adult.
7. Remolding is not limited by age but does contain elements of priority and time. Using molding in elderly patients can be remarkable.
8. Tissue changes in response to the Tidal Forces are different from reflexes modulated by the central nervous system. We are not in touch with a reflex world.
9. Facilitation in the central nervous system, spinal cord, and genes is a precursor to disease. The Tide works directly to quiet this process and modify it.
10. Nurture homeostasis.

RECIPROCAL TENSIONS

As Osteopathic physicians, we have all become familiar with the sensory experience of palpating the reciprocal tension within the tissues of the body. Dr. Sutherland's idea of a reciprocal tension membrane lends itself to both palpatory and treatment techniques that reveal directly to the physician a world of fulcrums, balance, and limits. Within the cranium one can palpate a dural system that easily exposes its tensile phenomena and its "suspended automatically shifting fulcrum."

This fulcrum, named after its discoverer, William G. Sutherland, is located at the junction of the great vein of Galen and the straight sinus. Its Automatic Shifting is limited by Tidal Forces that control the physiological motion of the tissues. The organized osseous system has limits that support the Intrinsic motion of the central nervous system. This synchronized motion of bone, membrane, and central nervous system in turn supports the biochemical exchange within all the fluids of the body. This is, of course, fundamental to Osteopathic thinking.

As physicians skilled in the recognition of the normal tensile potency and its natural range of motion, we have consequentially become aware of unhealthy patterns reflected as inertial phenomena within the body. We have also become familiar with treatment techniques that will resolve the inertial phenomena if we can properly establish a new state of balance that replicates the suspended automatically shifting fulcrum of a healthy system. This new fulcrum has the quality of a neutral state of balance, which, when established in the inertial tissue, allows the forces from within, that is the self-correcting forces, to shift the inertial tensile forces through a neutral fulcrum back into a moving reciprocal tension. This newly established motion may or may not reach the perfect original fulcrum. The motion within this new fulcrum reflects a resolution of inertia but at the same time represents the acknowledgment and the limits of the needs of the entire matrix of the body's tension as a whole, so an ideal may or may not ever be reached. However, even in this somewhat compromised state, all physiological functions that were held static within the inertial pattern are now free to move and restore health to all the tissues of the body.

Our work, then, is often to find these inertial conditions and to find a neutral point or a fulcrum around which motion can be organized to reestablish health. Having understood this fundamental concept, we come to ask ourselves the questions about the therapeutic use of the fluid and the potency! As clearly stated by A. T. Still, our ability to assist in establishing health is limited by our ability to perceive normal function. All systems within the body function in ways that are beautifully similar, and what I would like to propose is that perhaps we can look at the fluid and the potency within the human body and apply exactly the same laws that we do to the reciprocal tension membranes. Perhaps we will discover that there is a suspended automatically shifting fulcrum in the fluid and in the potency.

William Sutherland once stated as a question, "Do you see the fulcrum of the fluctuation of the cerebrospinal fluid? Do you see the fulcrum in the fluctuation of cerebrospinal fluid? Do you see the point? Do you see the point?" Dr. Sutherland reflected frequently upon a fluid drive and a potency—a potency inherent within the fluid that carried within its natural laws an organizational power that had an uncanny but predictable ability to heal.

Many students, when they meet this concept of fluid and potency, get quite nervous and feel they do not know how to "get there" and become quite frustrated. Most of the students will stumble on the concept of fluid fluctuation, fluid drive, and potency and enter this simple world with many questions and many misconceptions. Often one hears, "I want to work more with the fluid or the potency but I cannot get there." If you have the ability to establish a neutral in the inertial tissue and the ability to see a change occurring, then you have seen the effects of the interaction of tissue, fluid, and potency as a unit of function through a fulcrum. If you have observed a Neutral carefully, you will see that it has to be related to all levels of function, including the most subtle generative forces.

We are going to look very slowly and very patiently at the fulcrums within the fluid and the potency. We are going to dismantle a unit of function and observe the separate processes at work. This will be an observational exercise that is designed to initiate separately the Neutral within the tissue, within the fluid, and within the potency so that we can see these qualities and witness the natural laws more clearly. The more we are able to separate these functions, the more we will be able to understand the intention of the Tidal Forces, either directly or indirectly, through our application of forces that engage it in conversation. At the same time, we must fully realize that when these fulcrums are synchronized we may experience uncanny results using almost subliminal forces that reflect to us almost no power whatsoever and yet yield results that border on the miraculous. It is these kinds of uncanny experiences, as Dr. Sutherland called them, that keep us as physicians in a field of humility that allows us to use the indirect but to be ready at all moments to surrender to the direct influence of the Breath of Life.

Before we begin our observations, it is important that we explore a little further this idea of reciprocal tension and expand it to include fluid and potency. As we have already discussed, the reciprocal tension membrane has certain qualities. We know that the reciprocal tension has limits. It has a proscribed range of influence and confines itself to geometric fields that we call anatomy. We also know that the reciprocal tensions within tissues have suspended automatically shifting fulcrums. In the cranium they shift directly around a point of potency called the Sutherland Fulcrum. As we go to the periphery, these suspended automatically shifting fulcrums represent the functional center of the notochord at the middle of the nucleus pulposus of each segment. We know that this Automatic Shifting and these fulcrums are organized in such a way as to allow the life to function as a unified whole.

Suppose, instead of saying reciprocal tension membrane, I said to you "reciprocal tension fluid," and you let this idea of reciprocal tension fluid sit on your mind and at the same time envision your experience with the reciprocal tension membrane. Reciprocal tension fluid.

PAUSE.

Would we not have a suspended automatically shifting fulcrum at the point of balance in the fluid?

Would we not have a fulcrum around which the potency of the fluid drive was able to manifest its hydraulic forces? The fluid fluctuation has limits in its range of motion, or fluctuation, and this range of fluctuation is usually limited by a tissue, but it may be limited by an electromagnetic field; in either case, the limits within the fluid fluctuations are constructed in such a way as to support the reciprocal tension in both the membrane and the potency. All of us, I hope, have at this point worked with the lateral fluctuation of the cerebrospinal fluid, which is self-limiting not only in its natural state but also in a state of excitation. We have also noticed that the potency within the fluid can pass through the fluid and the membrane, as seen when we use techniques that direct the Tide. We have seen that the potency of the fluid is limited by the functional limits of the organizational matrix of the body, which appears eventually as the more dense state of life we call anatomy. That is to say that the electromagnetic field in the potency can organize the fluid to such a point that a condensation takes place and a structure appears; this is the foundation of embryology and self-correcting mechanisms.

If we ask the same question about the potency, and if I say to you reciprocal tension potency, or if I say to you tensile potency, or reciprocal tensile potency or reciprocating tensile potency, and you think about the fluid and the membrane and their reciprocal tensions and you hold all of that in your mind, what do you come to?

PAUSE.

Could we not say that the concept we used for the reciprocal tension membrane and the reciprocal tension fluid could also apply to the tensile forces of the potency? The potency has a tensile quality. Potency is reciprocally balanced around a fulcrum, and it is limited in its geometric pattern of that system (anatomy). Potency, when used therapeutically, limits itself. Potency concentrates itself and its forces and will respond to the application of forces that place it in neutral or in a state where it is free to move. This Neutral can be established in the tensile inertia of a field within the potency; when we feel this inertia and this immobility containing the potency, we very often have the feeling that the tissue under our hand has condensed, that it is very, very dense, has lost its life force or has become living stone, or that its extracellular space has become static. The end effect is a feeling under our hands of a "withering field." In order to stay healthy, tissue must be irrigated but the fluid cannot be dead. Within the fluid there must be a life force, an entire biochemical electromagnetic world that is invisible to us and yet has shape and organization and reciprocal tension. This must be present within the fluid in order to supply the invisible matrix around which the molecular world can organize itself and maintain a satisfactory level of function and anatomical integrity. I think the thing that we most commonly lose sight of when we think about potency is that the potency is directly responsible for the shape of the human body. The human form originally is the by-product of reciprocal tensile potency that produces the architectural matrix of all bodily systems, including the biochemical, and represents the invisible creative intentions of the Master Mechanic.

All reciprocal tensions are limited. Nothing roams unleashed in the natural world. Natural limits created by reciprocal tensions maintain the design of the body. They also create the design of our biochemistry where we have limits in our blood pH and our potassium ion concentration. We have a range of motion through which our blood sugar is normal. This reciprocal tension that limits and guides gives us a division of labor within the body, and when healthy and organized as a single unit of function is a beautiful thing to behold. It is a silent thing that moves like the wind, that moves as naturally as all living creatures that are in their natural state. A huge elephant moving through the brush in the wilderness of Africa makes no sound.

When this mechanism is free to function, we have simultaneity, synchronicity, and stillness perceived as graceful motion. It is this graceful motion that allows us as Osteopathic physicians to acknowledge that the original matrix is expressing itself and that our task has been completed.

All living things, including man, live within a background that nurtures their need. From this background emerges a world of interdependence, filled with infinite expression balanced by reciprocal tension, and manifesting a similarity that all living things share. When we join this background as physicians, we find one Living World, undivided, profoundly ordered BUT SINGULAR! Man is triune, and to dismantle the unity is to bring inertia into our work.

The reciprocal tensions in fluid, membrane, and potency are a singular event and will forever remain so, regardless of our nearsightedness.

To learn about natural law we will, both in concept and in palpation, dismantle this wonderful and beautiful Unit of Function, but let us always remember that this dismantling is our attempt to develop safe, predictable, and intelligent diagnostic and therapeutic modalities for our patients. Our most essential responsibility is to trust in the Wisdom of the Whole of Life. We are human beings, equal and kindred to everyone that seeks our advice.

A NOTE FROM THE WEARY

It is with deep sadness that I even write this note.

Since the conception of this program, material has been finding its way into some Craniosacral programs. I have been watching this rape of Osteopathy with detailed and precise observation for a long time, hoping I was wrong. I am absolutely sure that this mass exodus of material is done without any respect for our profession, the authorship, or for boundaries that are so important in Life.

The material here is an original creative work of my undertaking, and while I am acutely aware of the Source and lives that have nurtured it, I have been given the responsibility of organizing and designing the method in the light of the present course of the profession.

All aspects, including the language, are copyrighted and protected by laws. This obviously does not mean anything to those who take without any conscience. But ... it is not about legality ... it is about respect for traditions and their intrinsic value and boundaries. It is about practicing Osteopathic medicine without proper training.

I see clearly that deception is a skill that is being admired in today's world... sadly, we are all human and must be aware of ourselves... self-awareness is now being replaced by ideology, and, unfortunately, some people do not mind using "Stolen Goods."

Osteopathy is not a prostitute for the meaninglessness that others find in their lives that leads to cleverness and deception of their students. I am part of humanity, and as one member I am sad that we lack such understanding as the Tide wants from us. To become as Children we must be less clever than the adults around us.

This is my opinion from the last twenty-five years of watching and waiting and watching and listening and noticing books on Biodynamics from persons untrained in Osteopathy... what a contrast to my mentors ... who gave their lifeblood for the Health of this profession.

The human heart is very weak... It is our responsibility to be kind whenever possible ... I understand that the lesion at cause here is indwelling in us all... But we must grow up and be willing to lose it all rather than promote diluted skills that can be unhealthy for everyone.

We have a right to be a separate profession, and for good reason: it is great.

I promise you I will try to be as responsive as is possible.

I could not write this until I was free of anger and polarization ... that has taken years.

James Jealous, D.O., circa 2011

There is more, more than my lifetime can hold, but to those who love Osteopathy, I have written this for you, and no one else ... Thank you!

BIODYNAMICS OF OSTEOPATHY BOOK SERIES

This book is one of a series of twelve *Biodynamics of Osteopathy* books. It is recommended that you read the whole series in order, as each book builds on the understanding from prior books. It is also recommended that you seek experienced teachers and mentors to help you experience the full depth of the information given.

The full series is as follows:

Phase One is about involuntary motion, which is motion present in the whole and in the lesion. We learn to synchronize with the breathing of Primary Respiration before we approach any treatment. This synchronization is the key to working with stable rates and not irritating the system. The principle of synchronizing with a healthy aspect of the patient suffuses the whole teaching program. This synchronization shifts our awareness to a different level of receptivity, which allows us to see Primary Respiration rather than the lesion field, and this eventually leads us to an understanding of the intention of Primary Respiration.

Phase Two is about communication with the natural laws of healing that surround activity at 2 to 3 cycles per minute. We synchronize with the breathing of Primary Respiration and also add the skill of sensing the fulcrum, the Stillness through which the breathing creates form and function. It is a different kind of synchronization from that in Phase One, shifting our awareness more deeply. As this occurs, the treatment automatically expresses itself. The end point of treatment, when compared with Phase One, reveals several differences. We find this kind of synchronization works exclusively with the fluid body and the outcome of treatment is more complete than when working with tissue alone.

Phase Three is centered around the activities of the Long Tide (100 second cycle). We explore an indwelling therapeutic force already present in the lesion field. We learn that the dural system is not made-up of three sickles but rather a series of folds in a sac, arising during growth and development. We see the relationship between the upper and lower dural sacs, awakening us to the independence of two separate tentorium cerebelli. We discover that zone D, the horizon, and the Wire (along which the Long Tide moves during its intended therapeutic course) are all linked as natural laws pertaining to this level of Primary Respiration.

Phase Four focuses on the Midline, a place where the spatial relationships are expressed as a whole. It synchronizes and centers us in such a way that we become aware of Zone D and the Dynamic Stillness. The Third Level Stillness in Phase Four is different from the Stillness in the other Phases – we are centered by the Stillness at the center of creation. Our intention is replaced by the intention of the Tide which can facilitate our spiritual path.

Phase Five is about *the face*. As we approach the face, we use all of the principles that we have learned in Phase One, Two, Three, and Four. We work with automatic shifting and notice differences from how the face is viewed by older models within Osteopathy in the Cranial Field. As we synchronize with the therapeutic presence of the Long Tide we see what we can learn about the face from that landscape. We also work with Seams, Dynamic Stillness, and Ignition.

Phase Six is a continuation of our journey into the Wholeness that generates life and delivers therapeutic forces that transmute lesions once Neutral is expressed. It is a mixture of activities centered around the outside presence of Primary Respiration as something that is a non-biological force and that has a persona. We will also continue to explore seams and then move on to the extremities, first in the embryological terms and then as Sutherland taught them in his work called PowerPoints. Phase 6 is a time to build your understanding of the Tide and refine your skills.

Phase Seven highlights the Health. Dr. Still's famous comment "Find the Health; anyone can find disease," has plagued many minds over the last century. We come to the clear vision of several indwelling aspects of the Health: Love ... liquid light ... and a diamond matrix. A approach to the terminally ill and dying patient is addressed. In the somatic sensation of the Tide passing through the House Under the Sea, our awareness is transmuted by the Health. The lesion is seen as a precognitive act of the Health. Thoracic Respiration, Primary Respiration, and Ignition are as One. The landscape is vast ... and the principles of healing are even more substantial than we have previously experienced..

Phase Eight is a deeper exploration of seams, balanced rhythmic interchange, and the Flame of Intention as a therapeutic modality. Phase Eight is the culmination of our awareness of Wholeness, and ultimately brings us to the Divine Presence, Unconditional Love and Oneness. The living Tide dominates the awareness while forms move to the background. One feels the Breath of Creation in oneself as the Center of Wholeness. One feels the Unfoldment of oneself as one is Created. Our consciousness is a gift; we do not own it and if we try to control it we lose Wholeness.

Phase Nine is when we are able to fully evaluate and treat the Central Nervous System and the Eye. We also address Fire and the therapeutic modality of the Shakedown. True action is moved from Love and makes our perception exist. This Love is self-emptying and by its nature allows us to Serve as part of the Perfect. Perception can be used to Serve something other than ourselves. We have attempted to enter this balance point between the Perfect and the Disease ... it is a point where the whole of everything is suspended by Love as it works to incarnate the Complete. In the balance point of everything is The Intention of the Tide following the movement of the distortion back to a True relationship with the Blueprint of Life.

Pediatrics One explores how children grow as a whole, not in parts as we sometimes believe. Children live in the Direction of Ease of motion present in their fluid metabolic fields, otherwise they get uncomfortable and require assistance. Does your treatment directly support the whole, or does it assume to support the whole? We realize children are not adults and cannot be treated as adults are. We approach the therapeutic modality of the "Meeting Place", prenatal and postnatal periods, the treatment of the pelvis during pregnancy, fetal malposition and labor.

Pediatrics Two is where we deepen in the perceptive awareness necessary to approach the treatment of children. We deepen in our appreciation of Wholeness, the three levels of Stillness and the "Meeting Place". We approach "Desert Neutral", where therapeutics pass into the neutral substance, and a mystery unfolds as the breath of Divine love cascades as a therapeutic force across a night desert landscape, filling and leaving behind no visible effects. We further address treatment of the pelvis and the uterus during pregnancy. We explore thoracic and Primary Respiration in children, and the Family Circle.

Pediatrics Three is where we continue to study the therapeutic Flow of Attention. We deepen in Third Level Stillness and the Meeting Place. The Meeting Place is easily misinterpreted ... our observer must be so still and neutral that the process can be seen as it happens. The central nervous system in the child can be finally approached for evaluation and treatment. We explore teething and also the "locked up head". We use the therapeutic modality of the Flame of Intention, and its connection to the Breath of Life. Everything is transparent to the Breath of Life.

ABOUT THE AUTHOR

James Jealous, D.O. (1943–2021), was an osteopathic physician, teacher, and writer. His life's work was founding and developing **Biodynamics of Osteopathy**, a unique methodology he established within the field of osteopathy, following the lineage of Dr. A.T. Still and Dr. W.G. Sutherland.

He was born in Saco, Maine, and since his father was an osteopathic physician, he was around osteopathy from an early age. He studied at Kirksville College of Osteopathic Medicine in Missouri (now the A.T. Still University of Health Sciences), graduating in 1970. He then set up practice in rural Maine as an osteopathic primary care physician.

Over time, Dr. Jealous saw parallels between the work of embryologist Dr. Erich Blechschmidt and that of osteopathic physician Dr. William Garner Sutherland. This inspiration led him to create his own body of work. In the early 1990s, he began teaching "A Biodynamic View of Osteopathy in the Cranial Field," which, as he developed his specific methodology, was refined to "Biodynamics of Osteopathy."

A deeply spiritual person, he felt most at home in the natural world and was an avid fisherman and hiker.

For more information, please visit:
https://BiodynamicsOfOsteopathy.com

There is a wind passing through …
it is the motion of creation,
the eternal motion of Divine love.

www.ingramcontent.com/pod-product-compliance
Lightning Source LLC
LaVergne TN
LVHW071338210926
848486LV00003B/176

* 9 7 9 8 2 9 5 5 3 8 9 9 5 *